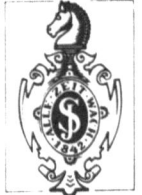

John Nicholls · Richard Glass

Coloproctology

Diagnosis and Outpatient Management

Foreword by John Alexander-Williams

With 49 Line Drawings by Geoffrey Lyth

Springer-Verlag
Berlin Heidelberg New York Tokyo

John Nicholls, MChir, FRCS
Consultant Surgeon,
St. Thomas' and St. Mark's Hospitals, London, UK.

Richard Glass, MS, FRCS
Senior Surgical Registrar,
The London Hospital, Whitechapel, London, UK.

Nicholls, R. J. Coloproctology: diagnosis and outpatient management
Includes bibliographies and index.
1. Proctology. 2. Colon (Anatomy) – Diseases. 3. Ambulatory medical care. I. Glass,
Richard, 1948–   . II Title [DNLM: 1. Colonic Diseases. 2. Rectal Diseases.
WI 520 N615c]
RC864.N53 1985 616.3'5 85–2808
ISBN-13: 978-3-540-15140-1   e-ISBN-13: 978-1-4471-1375-1
DOI: 10.1007/ 978-1-4471-1375-1

©by Springer-Verlag Berlin Heidelberg 1985

The use of registered names, trademarks, etc. in this publication does not imply, even
in the absence of a specific statement, that such names are exempt from the relevant
protective laws and regulations and therefore free for general use.

Product Liability: The publisher can give no guarantee for information about drug
dosage and application thereof contained in this book. In every individual case the
respective user must check its accuracy by consulting other pharmaceutical literature.

Filmset by Wenden Typesetting Services Limited, Saffron Walden, Essex.

2128/3916–543210

Foreword

In this age of specialization most patients with diseases of the hind gut and anus are still managed by general physicians or surgeons.

The speciality of coloproctology has grown from the art of 'anology', a study of conditions limited to that distance from the anal verge that could be inspected easily by torch- or candlelight or with the aid of a simple speculum. Two centuries ago many proctological ills were often treated by itinerant quacks, partly because the physician considered himself rather too grand to meddle around the anus and the medical profession in general tended to look down on those who studied anal disease.

Today, in certain countries, coloproctology has become a speciality every bit as exclusive as urology or orthopaedic surgery, with its own training programme and examinations, usually undertaken after the end of general surgical training. Such super-specialization has undeniable advantages with rapidly advancing technology and therapeutic possibilities. There is no doubt that for the patient suffering from a low rectal carcinoma or severe inflammatory bowel disease there are advantages in being treated by surgeons who are dealing with several cases in a year rather than by a general surgeon who sees such problems relatively rarely. Such specialized colorectal surgery units makes good sense medically and economically in large centres of population with good communications.

In the world at large, however, even including many parts of Europe and America, anorectal disease will continue to be assessed and treated by surgeons and physicians whose post-graduate training has been broadly based. In the course of a year such a practitioner may have to treat four or five cases of prolapsing haemorrhoids, twice as many of pruritus ani and one or two of anorectal sepsis. He or she may have to evaluate twenty patients with bright red rectal bleeding and two or three with bloody diarrhoea. This is not enough work to justify establishing a special unit, but it is vitally important work for the community, which deserves the very best of modern care and management. The community rightly expects its generalist physicians and surgeons to be of the highest standard, yet they cannot undergo extensive post-graduate training in every speciality nor attend every post-graduate course.

Those who deal with even a few colorectal and anal lesions each year can equip themselves with this handy textbook of coloproctology. Although it is essentially geared to outpatient management and assessment and is aimed at the doctor practitioner in a rectal clinic, it contains sufficient up-to-date information about all large bowel and anal diseases to give a firm grounding, even though it deliberately gives no operative details. Some might say that the general surgeon should not undertake such operative procedures as rectopexy, post-anal repair or low anterior resection and some would say that general surgeons should not undertake restorative proctocolectomy or ileo-anal procedures. Those who perforce have to, must study the most modern original articles or refer to surgical and technical encyclopaedias. All surgeons and physicians dealing with the assessment and primary treatment of disease of the distal large bowel need to be equipped with this book.

Birmingham, 1985   John Alexander-Williams
                                                    MD, ChM, FRCS, FACS

Preface

A major part of general surgery and gastroenterology involves the treatment of diseases of the colon and rectum—so much so that the rectal clinic has become a feature of many hospitals and colorectal surgery has now been accepted as a speciality. There are many detailed reference books dealing with diseases of the anus, rectum and colon, but a more practical approach to their diagnosis and management in the outpatient department could be helpful.

The book has been written in an attempt to assist young surgeons and physicians in training. It is aimed both at those for whom colorectal disease is included in a general surgical or gastroenterological education and at those who will confine themselves chiefly to anal problems. Emphasis is placed on essential aspects of diagnosis, assessment and treatment of patients in the outpatient department. Inpatient management is referred to only where it might influence the outpatient consultation and details of operative technique are avoided unless the procedure can be carried out in the rectal clinic.

The management of colorectal disease has advanced considerably in the last 10 years and the book has embraced progress by putting it in the context of modern practice. The book's form has forced the authors to be didactic, but references to recent publications have been offered as a guide to further reading.

The authors would like to thank Miss J. Grimsey and Miss D. Tolfree for their help with the manuscript.

London, 1985   John Nicholls
                                                                Richard Glass

Contents

1 The Rectal Clinic

Facilities

Diagnosis and successful treatment of diseases of the anus, rectum and colon depend to a considerable extent on a well-run outpatient department. This should provide a suitable examination suite, adequate equipment and efficient nursing.

Much depends on the nurse in charge, who should be responsible for the co-ordination of patient movement within the clinic, the delegation of duties to her nurses, and the immediate administration of notes, investigation requests and biopsy specimens. It is clearly preferable if the nurses are long-standing members of the department, but this may be difficult in teaching hospitals, where they tend to move from one appointment to another after a few weeks. The nurses should understand the nature of the diseases encountered and their treatment, be able to position patients correctly, look after equipment and be ready to receive biopsy and stool specimens. At least two nurses should be instructed in the cleaning, care and simple maintenance of the flexible sigmoidoscope. Commitment can be encouraged by showing the nurses lesions and allowing them to look down endoscopes.

The general arrangement of the rectal clinic must offer privacy for the patient and adequate heating. The basic requirements are a waiting area, examination rooms with at least one adjacent changing room each, a wash area for cleaning instruments, a sluice, an area for the sister and at least two lavatories. Flexible sigmoidoscopy requires bowel preparation by a disposable enema and usually takes several minutes to perform. It is therefore preferable to set aside for this examination a separate endoscopy room, which should also be equipped with a sink and draining board and have space for cleaning and storing the equipment. In many hospitals there is an endoscopy room in the outpatient department suite.

Equipment

An examination couch with a firm surface sufficiently high for the examiner to sit comfortably is essential. Special proctological tables are available. The Ritter examination couch (Ritter, USA) has an electrically operated hydraulic raise-and-tilt mechanism and can be broken in two places to accommodate a modified knee–elbow position. Special tables with leg attachments for lithotomy position examinations are also available (Wolfe, West Germany).

Two trolleys should be available, the first for equipment for digital examination and rigid sigmoidoscopy and proctoscopy (Fig. 1.1) and the second for equipment for flexible sigmoidoscopy (Fig. 1.2). Trolley 1 should be placed at the foot of the examination couch within easy reach of the examiner. Trolley 2 can either be placed on one side and moved to the couch when flexible sigmoidoscopy is performed or kept in the endoscopy room.

A sucker is needed, particularly if the bowel is prepared before examination since the rectum often contains liquid from the enema.

Rigid Sigmoidoscopes

Rigid sigmoidoscopes can have either distal or proximal lighting. The former type has the disadvantage that the bulb may become coated with faeces. The various

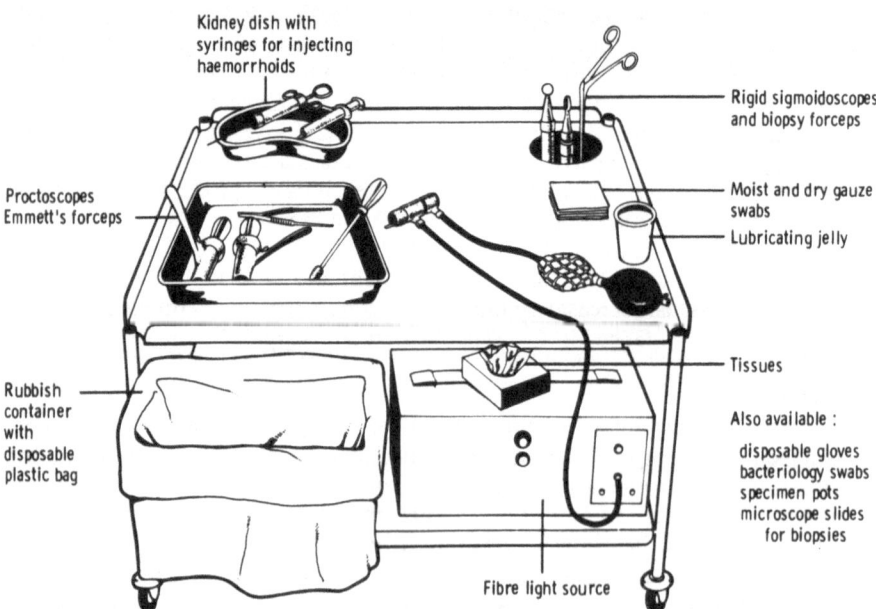

Fig. 1.1. Equipment for digital examination, rigid sigmoidoscopy and proctoscopy.

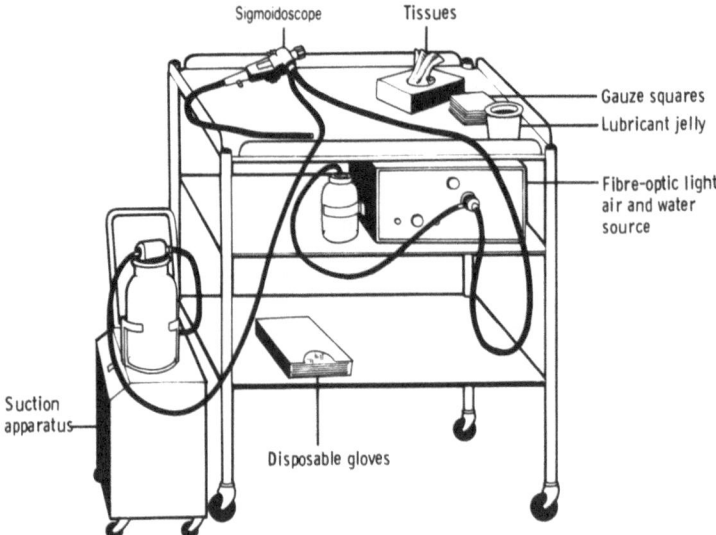

Fig. 1.2. Equipment for flexible sigmoidoscopy.

designs of sigmoidoscopes with proximal lighting all have certain common features. Lloyd Davies's pattern is shown in Fig. 1.3 and is excellent for routine use. Various lengths and diameters are available but the 25 cm long instrument of 15 mm bore is most satisfactory for general work. A wider bore (20 mm) instrument 20 cm long enables a more detailed examination of the rectum, but is more uncomfortable for the patient. The paediatric sigmoidoscope with a diameter of 9 mm may be useful in adults with painful anal lesions since it is almost always possible to introduce this smaller instrument into the rectum without exacerbating pain.

A fibre-optic lighting system is preferable to a battery-powered arrangement. It is more reliable and the intensity of light is greater. Bulbs and the fibre-optic flex may need replacing from time to time; the life expectancy of the latter is diminished by twisting or kinking, which fracture fibres in the bundle. Unless well maintained, battery systems often fail owing to faulty connections in the wiring and a tendency for bulbs to blow if the current is increased too rapidly on adjusting the rheostat. They can, however, be used where no power socket is available.

Biopsy forceps with trephine cusps of both elongated and rounded shape should be available. The Patterson and Chevalier Jackson models (Fig. 1.3) are suitable examples of each type. Besides being used for taking biopsies, they can also hold small gauze swabs for cleaning the lumen down the sigmoidoscope. An alternative method of cleaning the sigmoidoscope is to use specially prepared disposable cotton wool swabs mounted on long sticks.

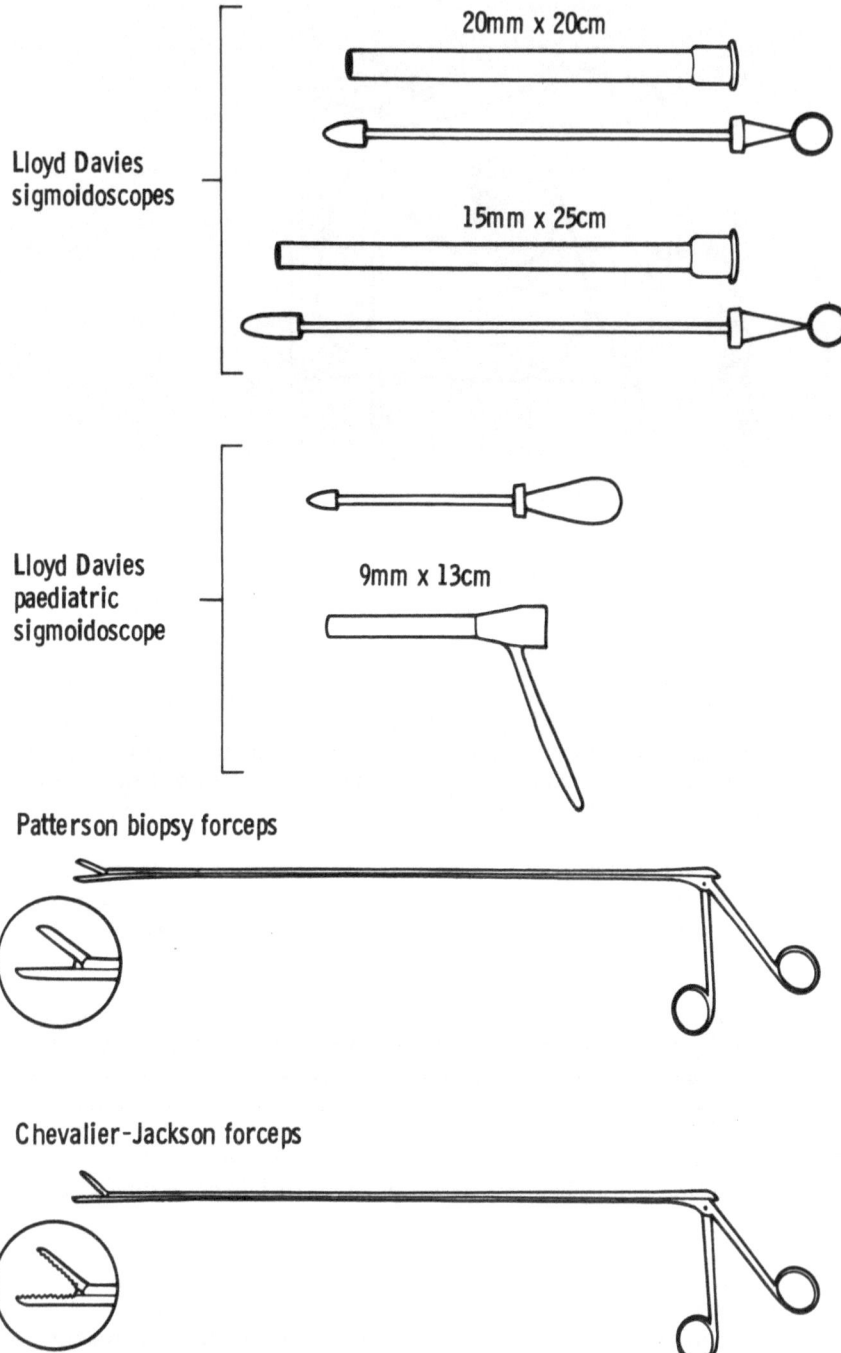

Fig. 1.3. Rigid sigmoidoscopes and biopsy forceps.

Equipment

Proctoscopes (Fig. 1.4)

The bigger the proctoscope which can be passed, the better the view obtained. For general use the type of instrument designed by Naunton-Morgan is suitable; it measures 7 cm in length and 21 mm in diameter, and affords a transverse view of the lower rectum and anal canal. In addition it is essential to have a

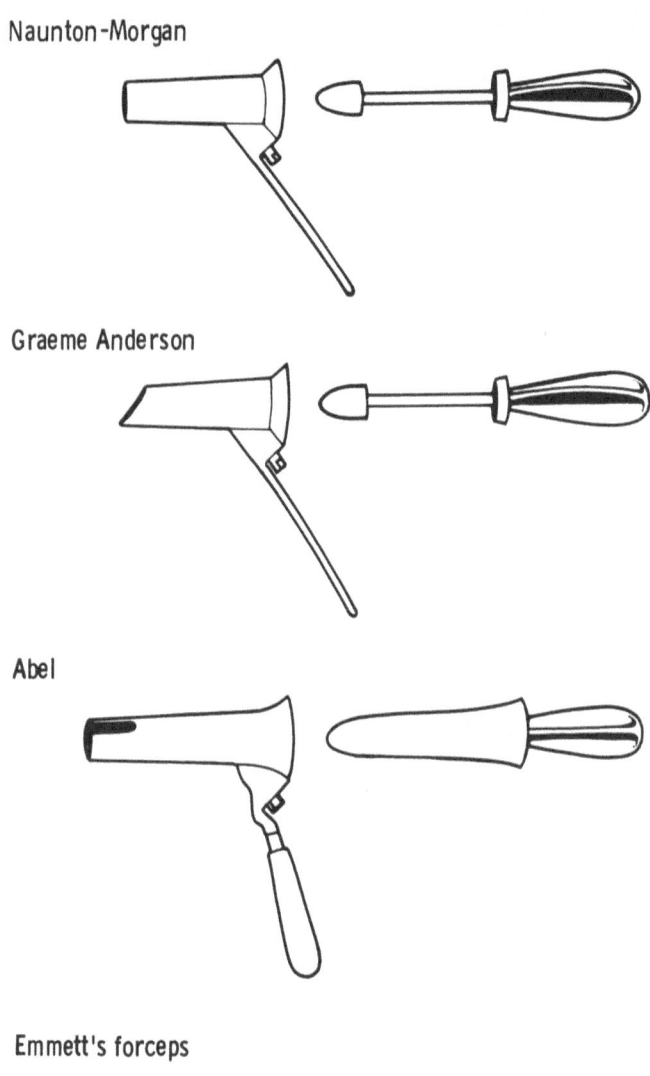

Naunton-Morgan

Graeme Anderson

Abel

Emmett's forceps

Fig. 1.4. Proctoscopes and Emmett's forceps.

proctoscope which will give an oblique view of the anal canal. The Graeme Anderson proctoscope has a bevelled end and is particularly useful when searching for the internal openings of fistulas or assessing the healing of surgical wounds in the ánal canal. The Abel proctoscope (Thackerey) has a 3 cm slot cut into the side that allows mucosa and haemorrhoidal tissue to bulge into the lumen of the instrument, which is useful for injection sclerotherapy.

Illumination provided by a fibre-optic source is excellent but it is usually adequate ànd more convenient to use an adjustable lamp (Anglepoise) at the foot of the couch. The lumen of the proctoscope can be cleaned by gauze swabs held on long non-toothed forceps such as Emmett's forceps. There is little place for adjustable anal specula in the outpatient department.

Flexible Sigmoidoscopes

It has been possible for many years to visualise the rectum and often the lower sigmoid colon by rigid sigmoidoscopy, but the introduction of the flexible sigmoidoscope has allowed the direct examination of the whole left side of the colon in many cases. This is a considerable advance since most colonic lesions arise in this part of the bowel.

Flexible sigmoidoscopes are made by all manufacturers of fibre-optic medical instruments. There are slight differences between the models—for example in length (60–75 cm) and in the flexibility of the shaft and the umbilical. The parts of a typical instrument are shown in Fig. 1.5. The instrument should be handled with care. The delicate fibre-optic bundle is damaged by kinking (which causes

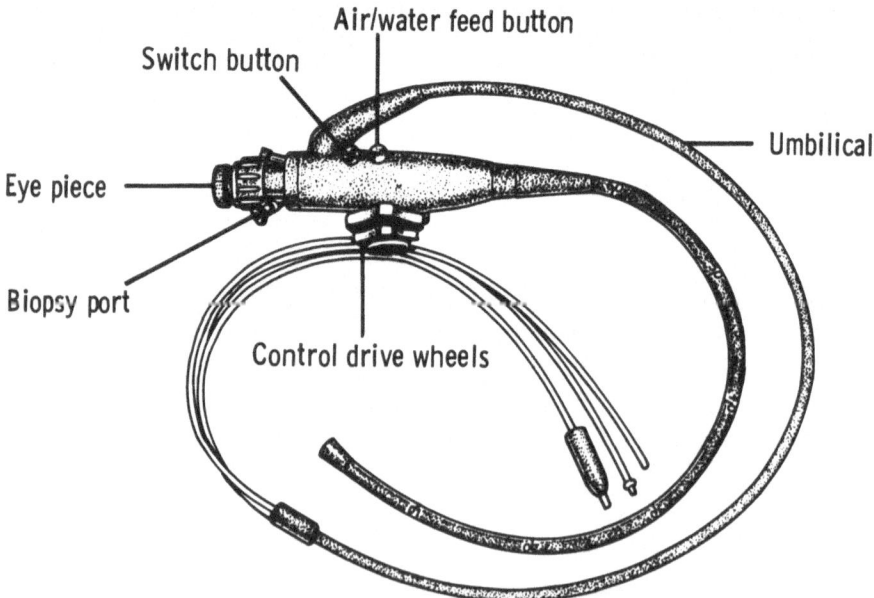

Fig. 1.5. Flexible sigmoidoscope: essential features.

fracture of the fibres), the wires from the drive wheels controlling movement of the tip may become strained with excessive angulation and poor cleaning will result in blocking of the channel. Most instruments are fitted with an automatic water feed, but some are not. Air supply and lighting are provided from a combined air/light source unit and a separate suction pump is available although any standard suction apparatus is satisfactory. Biopsy forceps, cleaning brushes and spare diaphragms for the biopsy port are also supplied. Teaching attachments and a camera are available too. Photography, however, requires a special high-intensity light source. Servicing can be arranged with the manufacturer's local agents and is advisable after every 100 examinations.

Miscellaneous Equipment

The following equipment should also be available.

Treatment of Haemorrhoids

Syringes with straight and angled needles for injection of sclerosant

Solutions for injection sclerotherapy (5% phenol in arachis oil, sodium tetradecate (Thrombovar))

Rubber band ligation set

Cryoprobe (optional)

Infrared coagulator (optional)

Specimens

Specimen pots containing formalin (10%) for biopsies

Sterile specimen pots for the collection of pus, faeces etc.

Bacteriological swabs and transport media

Dressings

Dressings and finger cots for the management of surgical wounds at home

Cleaning of Instruments

Metal instruments, including rigid endoscopes, must be thoroughly washed in antiseptic solution (e.g. cetrimide 1%) and rinsed in water. They should then be boiled for 5–10 minutes.

Thorough cleaning of the flexible sigmoidoscope is important to keep the channel and internal tubing of the instrument clear and to reduce bacterial colonisation to a minimum. It should be cleaned before starting the session and immediately after an examination. Water should be sucked through and the suction channel cleaned with a brush mounted on a wire introduced via the biopsy port. The biopsy port is unscrewed and cleaned and the shaft and channel are washed with a soap solution, exposed to a solution of glutaraldehyde (Cidex 2%) for 2–3 minutes and then washed in water and dried. This procedure must be carried out between each examination, and at the end of the clinic the shaft is immersed in glutaraldehyde for at least 10 minutes and washed and dried. Gloves must be worn to avoid contact with the glutaraldehyde, which can cause skin eruptions and irritation of mucous membranes. The head and umbilical of the instrument should not come into contact with water or antiseptic agents, but can be cleaned with alcohol (70%).

Minor Operations

Certain surgical procedures can be performed in the rectal clinic; these include excision of skin tags, excision or drainage of a perianal varyx and drainage of abscesses. The authors feel that sphincterotomy for anal fissure should be carried out under general anaesthetic, perhaps as a day case procedure, but accept that many surgeons consider local anaesthesia satisfactory.

Instruments

Good illumination and well-kept surgical instruments are necessary. The practice of supplying the rectal clinic with rejects from the main operating theatre should be discouraged as the circumstances of an outpatient procedure may not be ideal and blunt or unsuitable instruments only add to any difficulty. Many more outpatient procedures would probably be performed if adequate facilities and equipment were available.

The necessary instruments are shown in Fig. 1.6. For obtaining exposure for intra-anal procedures the Eisenhammer anal speculum is recommended. It is easy to introduce and remove and gives excellent access.

Fine-toothed and non-toothed forceps, sharp-pointed scissors and a selection of absorbable sutures (for example plain catgut or Dexon (2/0)) should be available. A small needle holder, a pair of suture scissors and a fine probe complete the basic equipment.

Local Anaesthesia

Lignocaine (1%) is usually satisfactory as a local anaesthetic, although the surgeon may wish to use lignocaine with adrenaline in a concentration of 1:200 000 for its haemostatic effect. Lignocaine is a cardiac depressant and the

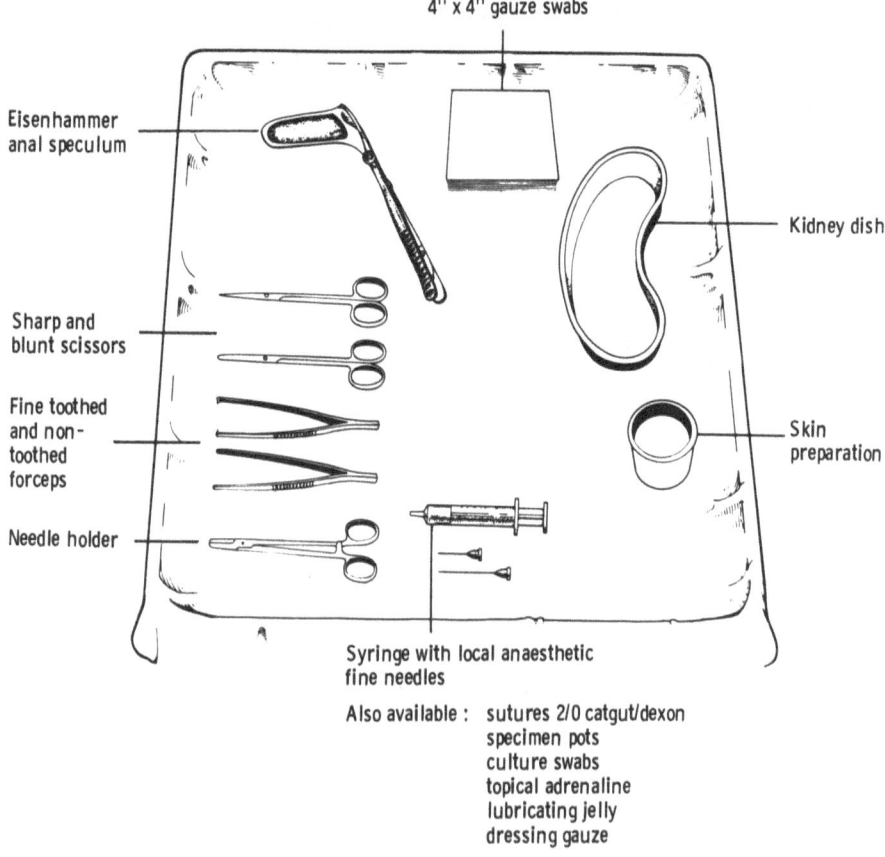

Fig. 1.6. Instruments required for minor anal operations.

dose is limited to 250 mg where plain local anaesthetic is used and to 400 mg where local anaesthetic is combined with adrenaline.

Local infiltration of 5–10 ml is satisfactory for small lesions. Where the procedure is more extensive (e.g. sphincterotomy) the additional injection of 10 ml of lignocaine into each ischiorectal fossa will give enhanced anaesthesia and relaxation of the anal sphincter by blockade of the inferior haemorrhoidal nerves.

Preparation

Written consent by the patient must be obtained. Preparation of the bowel by glycerine suppositories or a disposable phosphate enema is sufficient to empty the rectum.

Operations can be carried out with the patient in either the lithotomy or the left lateral position. In the latter case an assistant will be required to display the anus by traction on the upper buttock. Chlorhexidine (1%) in aqueous solution is a satisfactory skin preparation; under no circumstances should a spirit-based antiseptic be used.

Further Reading

Bouchier IAD, Allan RN, Hodgson HJF, Keighley MRB (eds) (1984) Textbook of gastroenterology. Baillière Tindall, London

Goldberg SM, Gordon PH, Nivatvongs S (1980) Essentials of anorectal surgery. Lippincott, Philadelphia

Goligher JC (1984) Surgery of the anus, rectum and colon. Baillière Tindall, London

Thomson JPS, Nicholls RJ, Williams CB (eds) (1981) Colorectal disease. Heinemann, London

2 Examination

Almost all conditions affecting the anus and rectum can be diagnosed on physical examination, and in many cases disease of the left colon can be identified by flexible sigmoidoscopy. The examination should be carried out in the following order:

General examination
Inspection and palpation of perineum
Anorectal examination
Rectal digital examination
Rigid sigmoidoscopy
Proctoscopy
Flexible sigmoidoscopy

Rigid and flexible sigmoidoscopy give only a partial examination of the large bowel and further investigation is required if there is suspicion of more proximal disease.

The results of the examination should be recorded systematically and it is helpful to use a prepared examination sheet along the lines of that shown in Fig. 2.1. Printed diagrams to record findings are useful.

General Examination

A general examination of the patient is important as many diseases of the large bowel, rectum and anus have systemic manifestations. Lymphadenopathy,

General Condition

Abdomen

Inguinal Lymph Nodes

Ano-rectal Examination

Inspection   Skin
                    Perineal descent
                    Anal reflex

Palpation   Sphincter resting tone
                    Voluntary contraction
                    Cough reflex
                    Levator wasting

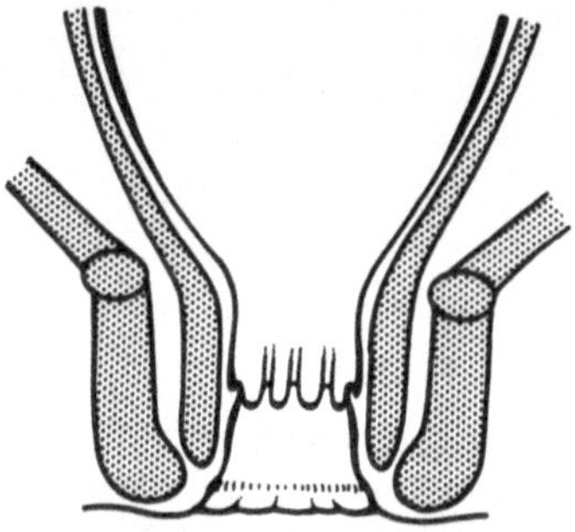

Sigmoidoscopy   To   cm

                    Biopsy at   cm

Proctoscopy

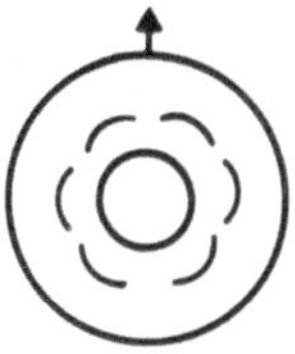

Flexible sigmoidoscopy   To   cm

                          Biopsies   cm

cm.
15
10
5
0

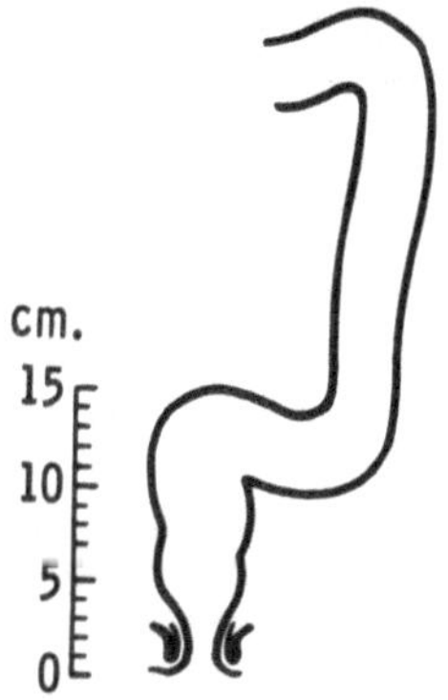

Fig. 2.1. Examination sheet.

anaemia, hepatic enlargement and abdominal masses and distension may occur in both malignant and inflammatory bowel disease. Lymph nodes, particularly in the supraclavicular and inguinal areas, should be examined. Inguinal lymphadenopathy may be present in anal carcinoma or anorectal sepsis. In inflammatory bowel disease arthropathy, uveitis, and skin lesions such as erythema nodosum and pyoderma gangrenosum and oral ulceration may develop; liver disease in the form of chronic hepatitis, cirrhosis or sclerosing cholangitis occurs in about 5% of cases. Clubbing of the finger nails is often seen in Crohn's disease.

Patients may be wasted and show signs of malnutrition. In the severely ill subject an assessment of the state of the circulation and of water and electrolyte depletion is essential. A general neurological examination may be relevant.

Anorectal Examination

Anorectal examination is everyday practice to the doctor but to patients it is an unusual event. Many are embarrassed and fear that it will be painful. The clinician's first task, therefore, is to gain the confidence of the patient. An unhurried demeanour, taking time to listen to the patient's story, explaining in advance the sequence of examination and what the patient may feel at each stage, help to allay anxiety. The room should be well heated and a small blanket covering the thighs may make the patient feel less exposed.

Position of the Patient

Three positions for the patient are in general use: the left lateral, the knee-elbow and the lithotomy. Although the choice is largely determined by the habit and training of the clinician there are advantages and disadvantages to each.

With the patient in the left lateral position inspection of the perineum, digital examination and sigmoidoscopy are simple and the patient can lie in a relaxed and comfortable attitude. This is an advantage, particularly with old or frail patients or when the examination is made at the bedside. Access for the clinician is excellent provided the patient is correctly placed, and procedures such as injection or rubber band ligation of haemorrhoids or rectal biopsy can be carried out with ease. Patients with pelvic floor disorders including rectal prolapse are best examined in the left lateral position since they can strain down or contract the sphincter without difficulty when asked to do so by the examiner.

The knee–elbow position gives an excellent view of the rectum and passage of the rigid sigmoidoscope past the rectosigmoid junction may be easier than with the left lateral position since the sigmoid colon tends to fall towards the anterior abdominal wall, straightening the rectosigmoid angle. The position is, however, uncomfortable for some patients and is generally less well tolerated than the left lateral position.

The lithotomy position gives an excellent view of the anterior perineum as well as the anus but a special table is required and assessment of the pelvic floor muscles may be difficult. It is, however, a suitable position for operative treatment of some conditions of the rectum, anus and perineum.

The left lateral position will be described in detail (Fig. 2.2). It helps to have nurses familiar with it and for whom arranging the patient correctly is second nature. Positioning starts with the patient sitting up. He or she then turns to the left and rests the point of the left elbow on the far edge of the couch. With the weight of the body supported by the left elbow and leg, the patient raises the buttocks; the nurse, by placing her left arm under the patient, can then grip the left hip and gently bring the buttocks towards her to project about 10 cm beyond the near edge of the couch. A small sandbag slipped under the left buttock raises the pelvis. The patient's trunk should lie at 45 degrees to the long axis of the couch and the head, resting on a pillow, should be level with its far edge. The hips are flexed and the feet placed level with the far edge of the couch, with about 120 degrees of flexion at the knees.

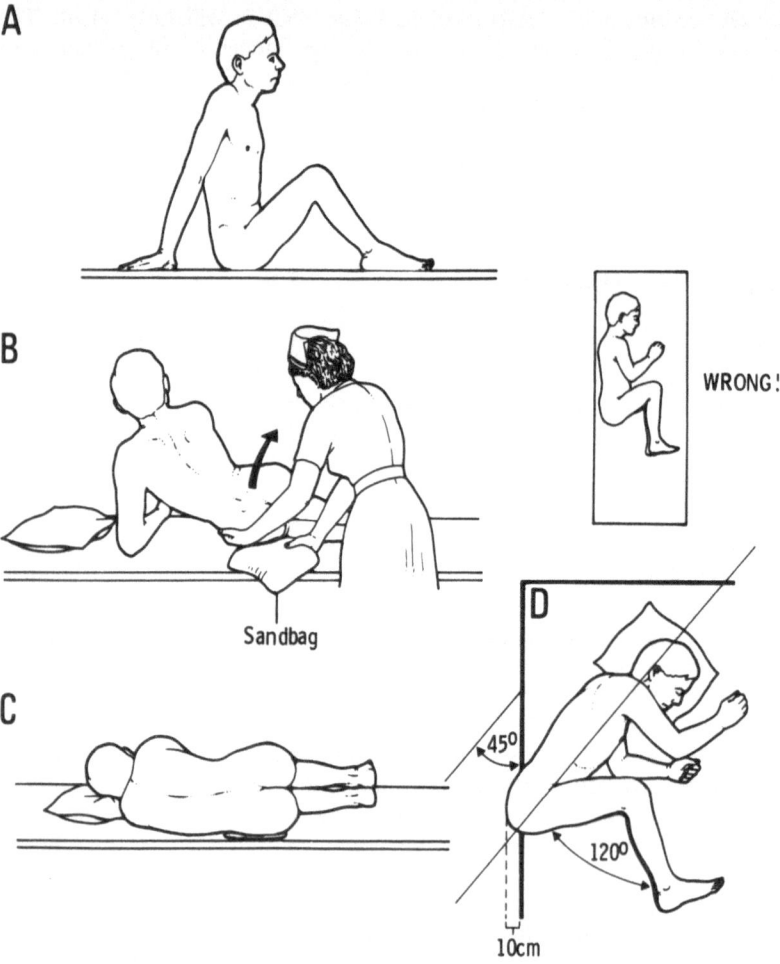

Fig. 2.2. Anorectal examination: the left lateral position.

Inspection (Fig. 2.3)

The normal anus is oval with its long axis lying sagittally. There is often some laxity of the perianal skin but the circumferential groove between the internal and external sphincters can often be seen as a surface marking in a thin patient.

Several conditions can be diagnosed entirely on inspection, including dermatoses, some abscesses and fistulas, prolapsing haemorrhoids, rectal prolapse, hidradenitis suppurativa, anal tumours, pilonidal sinus and sexually transmitted diseases such as condylomata acuminata, syphilitic lesions and herpes.

a) Direct inspection

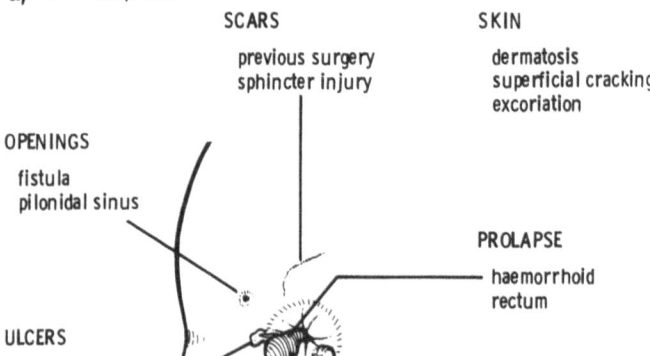

SCARS
previous surgery
sphincter injury

SKIN
dermatosis
superficial cracking
excoriation

OPENINGS
fistula
pilonidal sinus

PROLAPSE
haemorrhoid
rectum

ULCERS
fissure (tag)
Crohn's
chancre

LUMPS
varyx
tags
tumour
warts

Fig. 2.3a–c. Inspection: possible abnormalities.

The presence of moisture, pus, mucus, blood and faecal soiling should be noted and the perianal skin then gently parted (Fig. 2.3b). This may reveal lesions lying in the lower anal canal—such as a fissure, which is usually found in the midline posteriorly or anteriorly. Laxity of the anal orifice suggests weakness of the anal sphincter and may indicate an underlying rectal or mucosal prolapse, faecal impaction or weakness of the pelvic floor. Scars indicating previous trauma (including operations) may be an important clue to the diagnosis.

The patient is then asked to strain to demonstrate any prolapsing haemorrhoids, prolapse of the rectum, faecal leakage or abnormal perineal descent (Fig. 2.3c). Normally the anal orifice lies about 2–3 cm above the ischial tuberosities. If, at rest, it lies level with the ischial tuberosities or, on straining, descends more than 1 cm below them, abnormal pelvic floor descent can be inferred. This is more marked when the patient strains while standing.

b) Parting the anus

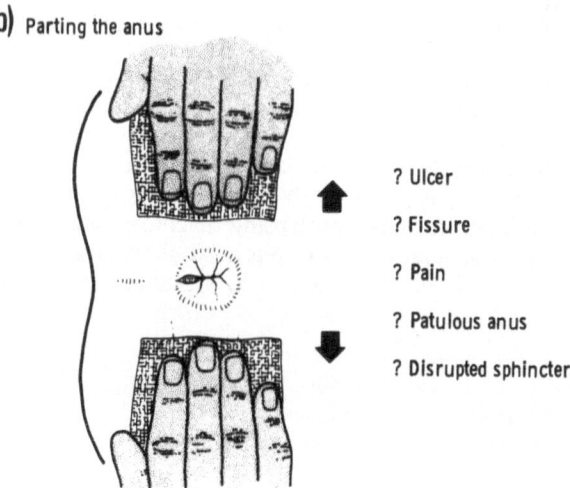

? Ulcer

? Fissure

? Pain

? Patulous anus

? Disrupted sphincter

c) Straining

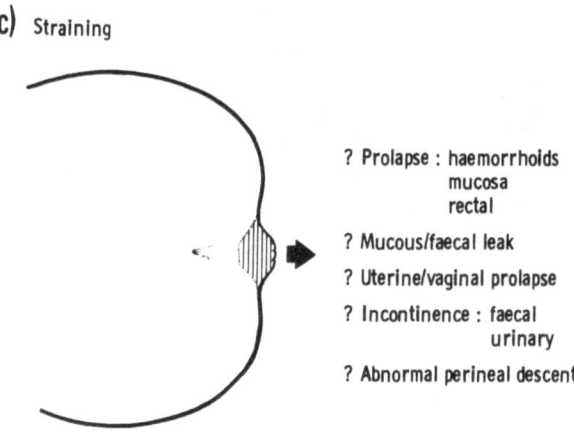

? Prolapse : haemorrhoids
                  mucosa
                  rectal

? Mucous/faecal leak

? Uterine/vaginal prolapse

? Incontinence : faecal
                     urinary

? Abnormal perineal descent

Palpation of the Perianal Region (Fig. 2.4)

Palpation of the perianal region and natal cleft is done systematically from the anal verge outwards. The tip of the coccyx lies about 2–3 cm behind the anal orifice, the ischial tuberosities on each side and the scrotum or vulva in front. The intersphincteric groove is often palpable.

Fissures, abscesses and a thrombosed perianal varyx are tender in the acute phase. An abscess may be difficult to identify if the lesion is deeply placed but a

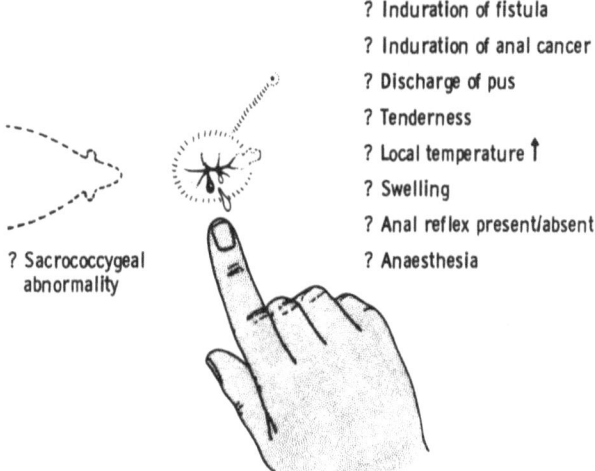

? Induration of fistula

? Induration of anal cancer

? Discharge of pus

? Tenderness

? Local temperature ↑

? Swelling

? Anal reflex present/absent

? Anaesthesia

? Sacrococcygeal
abnormality

Fig. 2.4. Palpation.

thrombosed varyx produces a demarcated swelling just beneath the skin immediately adjacent to the anal orifice. Chronic abscesses and fistulas are surrounded by inflammatory infiltration which produces hardness of the tissues (referred to as induration). Induration is felt around external openings and may be felt as a cord beneath the skin indicating the site and direction of a track. A carcinoma feels hard.

In patients with symptoms of faecal incontinence or of prolapse a neurological examination of the perianal region is essential. This consists of testing the anal reflex and perianal sensation and should be performed before rectal digital examination or instrumentation. Firm stroking or pinching of the perianal skin produces a brisk involuntary contraction of the external sphincter seen as a twitch of the perianal skin on the same side as the stimulus. The reflex should be tested on both the right and left sides of the anus. A reduction or absence of the reflex indicates a lesion anywhere in the spinal reflex arc from sensory receptors in the anal skin to the muscle fibres of the external sphincter via the second, third or fourth sacral spinal segments. The perianal skin is supplied by sensory nerves of the third, fourth and fifth sacral segments. Anaesthesia in this area may indicate a spinal or cauda equina lesion. A general examination of the nervous system must be made when neurological disease is suspected.

Rectal Digital Examination (Fig. 2.5)

Rectal digital examination should be carried out methodically, carefully palpating the rectal mucosa, the rectal wall and extrarectal structures. A suitable order of

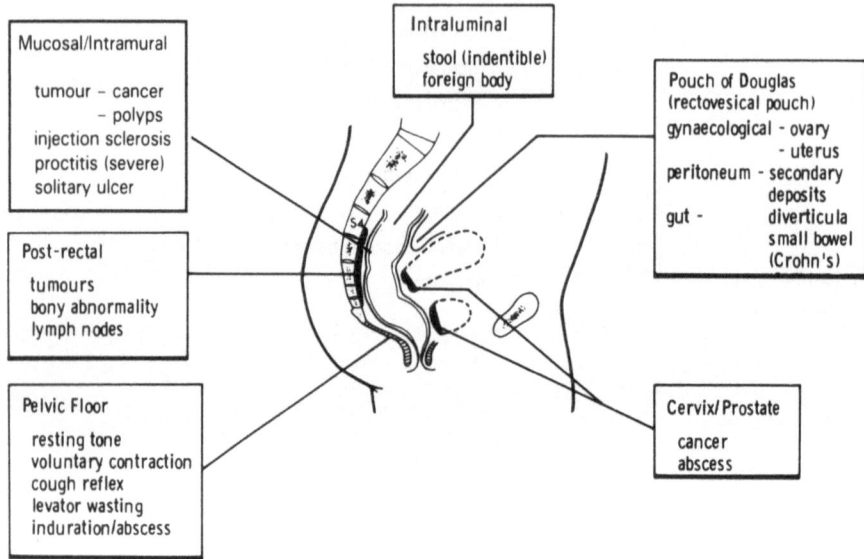

Mucosal/Intramural

tumour – cancer
       – polyps
injection sclerosis
proctitis (severe)
solitary ulcer

Intraluminal

stool (indentible)
foreign body

Pouch of Douglas
(rectovesical pouch)
gynaecological - ovary
             - uterus
peritoneum - secondary
             deposits
gut -   diverticula
             small bowel
             (Crohn's)

Post-rectal

tumours
bony abnormality
lymph nodes

Pelvic Floor

resting tone
voluntary contraction
cough reflex
levator wasting
induration/abscess

Cervix/Prostate

cancer
abscess

Fig. 2.5. Rectal digital examination.

examination is to feel the rectum first, other pelvic structures second, the pelvic floor third and the anal canal last.

The pulp of the right index finger is pressed gently against the anus and when the sphincter begins to give, the finger is slightly flexed and passed into the rectum. It is then advanced as far as possible.

Rectum

The average index finger can examine the rectum up to 10–12 cm from the anal verge when the knuckles of the hand are pressed into the perineum, except in individuals with a deep natal cleft and muscular buttocks. The finger initially passes posteriorly towards the coccyx and then runs upwards along the sacral concavity. The valves of Houston are encountered and as the finger advances it should be swept in a circular manner around the lumen, systematically palpating the mucosa, which is normally smooth.

Extrarectal Structures

In both sexes the coccyx and concavity of the sacrum up to about the third sacral segment are felt posteriorly. The lateral pelvic wall can be felt in its lower part as it becomes continuous with the levator ani muscle on each side.

In the male the prostate lies anteriorly, extending from about 6 to 8 cm above the anal verge. The smooth lateral lobes and midline sulcus can easily be felt.

Above the prostate a loop of bowel in the rectovesical pouch is sometimes palpable, particularly if it is loaded with faeces. In the female the cervix is felt as a firm mobile structure anterior to the rectum. The uterus can often be felt bimanually. The recto-uterine pouch of Douglas, lying above the cervix, may normally contain a retroverted uterus, an ovary or loop of bowel.

Pelvic Floor

The finger is then brought down onto the levator ani muscle on each side, and to the anorectal ring which is identified by the puborectalis sling. It is helpful when palpating these structures to apply the thumb to the perianal skin to act as counterpressure to the index finger. This enables muscle bulk and tone, both at rest and on voluntary contraction, to be assessed more precisely than is possible with the index finger alone. In normal individuals the ischio- and ileococcygeal components of the levator ani can be felt on each side as bulky contractile structures extending to the lateral pelvic wall.

The puborectalis can be palpated posteriorly and on both sides as a prominent sling passing round the gut tube, but is absent anteriorly. Besides marking the anorectal junction it creates an angle between the rectum and anal canal which is normally about 90 degrees. The size of the anorectal angle can be roughly assessed by estimating the directions of the anal canal and the lower rectum with the finger hooked over the puborectalis sling. Contraction of the puborectalis causes the sling to move anteriorly. Involuntary contraction of the pelvic floor can be induced by coughing (cough reflex); this indicates whether normal stretch reflexes are intact and allows anal canal tone at rest and during voluntary contraction to be estimated. About 60%–80% of resting pressure is due to contraction of the involuntary internal sphincter while the external sphincter is entirely responsible for the increase in pressure during voluntary contraction.

Anal Canal

The anal canal extends from the anorectal junction marked by the puborectalis to the anal verge. It is inclined towards the umbilicus and is about 3–4 cm long. The contour of the anal canal is smooth, with no normally palpable features. Lesions of the anal canal should be palpated between finger and thumb since this enables a more accurate assessment of their size and site.

After withdrawal the finger must be inspected for blood, mucus, pus and the colour of the stool. Blood or mucus may be signs of inflammatory bowel disease and neoplasm. Melaena or a pale stool may be clues to upper intestinal disease.

Vaginal Examination

A vaginal examination should be carried out whenever associated gynaecological disease or anorectal pathology involving the female organs or pelvis is suspected.

It must not be omitted in carcinoma of the rectum or where a mass is felt per rectum, since there may be involvement of the vagina, uterus or adnexae.

Abnormalities on Digital Examination

Rectum

A mass felt within the rectum may be due to a neoplasm, faeces or occasionally a foreign body. Benign neoplasms are soft and may therefore be difficult to feel. A neoplasm thought to be benign must be carefully palpated for hard areas indicating malignant change. A carcinoma is hard and usually ulcerated. Faeces are differentiated from a carcinoma by their indentibility. A cancer may or may not be mobile depending on the extent of local spread or of surrounding inflammatory reaction. The number of quadrants involved is an indication of the degree of local advancement and circumferential growths may cause stricturing of the lumen.

A solitary rectal ulcer may feel like a carcinoma if it is hard, and biopsy is needed to make the distinction. A submucous lipoma or fibroma is felt as a smooth mobile nodule covered by an intact mobile mucosa. The sclerosis that follows injection of haemorrhoids can cause induration and this may confuse the examiner if the history is not known.

In inflammatory bowel disease affecting the rectum, the mucosa often has a velvet-like feel owing to oedema. Ulceration itself is not palpable but inflammatory polyps may be felt. The rectum may be narrowed in long-standing inflammation with intramural fibrosis. A stricture is more likely in Crohn's disease than in ulcerative colitis. Similar signs may be found in other forms of proctitis, for example that due to irradiation.

Extrarectal Structures

An abnormal mass felt behind the rectum is most likely to be due to one of four conditions: dermoid cyst, sacral chordoma, skeletal tumour or rectal duplication. All are rare. The prostate gland, or at least its posterior surface, can be assessed by rectal examination. It may be smoothly enlarged in benign hypertrophy, but a craggy hard irregular prostate with some obliteration of the median sulcus indicates a carcinoma. A tender prostate suggests prostatitis.

A mass in the pouch of Douglas is a common finding; it may be uterine (carcinoma of the body, fibroids), ovarian (carcinoma, cyst, benign solid tumour) or an area of endometriosis. In common with the rectovesical pouch in the male, the pouch of Douglas may contain a tender loop of sigmoid colon affected by diverticular disease, peritoneal tumour deposits or a pelvic abscess. These will be felt as induration or a mass, tender or not according to the pathological condition.

In patients with rectal cancer an attempt should be made to feel for enlarged perirectal lymph nodes, perhaps indicating involvement by tumour. This manoeuvre is essential when considering the possibility of local treatment.

Pelvic Floor and Anal Canal

Signs that indicate weakness of the pelvic floor and sphincter include wasting of the levator ani, poor resting tone in the anal canal, poor voluntary contraction of the puborectalis and external anal sphincter, loss of the cough reflex and a widening of the anorectal angle. In cases of traumatic injury to the sphincter mechanism the site of scarring and location of contracting muscle should be carefully assessed since this is the most important guide to surgical repair.

Resting anal canal tone is increased in painful conditions of the anus, for example fissure or abscess. Where digital examination is impossible an examination under anaesthetic may be required to establish the cause. Resting anal tone is also increased in some patients with Hirschsprung's disease.

The internal opening of a fistula is felt as an area of localised induration most usually at the level of the dentate line in the midline. An anal carcinoma feels hard with an elevated edge and ulcerated centre. Fibrous anal polyps are usually pedunculated and may be difficult to feel owing to their mobility. Non-neoplastic ulceration of the anal canal is also difficult to feel and usually occurs in Crohn's disease. A fissure may be palpated and, if chronic, the edge sometimes feels indurated and a distal sentinel tag and proximal papilla are often present. A chronic intersphincteric abscess, a condition which is often missed, can be felt as a tender circumscribed nodule situated half-way along the anal canal, usually in the midline posteriorly. An anal stricture may be the result of previous anal surgery, Crohn's disease or carcinoma. Haemorrhoids are not usually palpable but may be if very large or thrombosed.

Endoscopy

Rigid Sigmoidoscopy

The term 'sigmoidoscopy' is an abbreviation for the more correct 'proctosigmoidoscopy'. In many people it may be impossible to negotiate the rectosigmoid junction with the rigid instrument. These patients will not, therefore, have had a 'sigmoidoscopy' at all.

Opinions differ on whether the bowel should be prepared. It is convenient if faeces are absent and preparation by a disposable enema is the routine practice in many units. However, this may remove important physical signs of disease such as blood or mucus in the lumen originating from a site beyond the range of the instrument and it also prevents an assessment of the consistency and colour of the stool and the opportunity to obtain a sizeable specimen for microbiology. When faeces do prevent an adequate examination, as occurs in 10%–20% of cases, a disposable enema can be given and the examination repeated.

Technique (Fig. 2.6)

For examination with the patient in the left lateral position, the examiner stands by the couch and lifts the patient's left buttock with his left hand. The end of the instrument is held in the right hand and the lubricated tip applied to the anus. It is then advanced with a gentle, steady movement aiming in the direction of the umbilicus and after 4–5 cm a fall in resistance indicates that the rectum has been entered (Fig. 2.6a). The obturator is withdrawn and the left hand takes the end of the instrument in an overhand grip. The light source and window attachment are inserted with the right hand which then holds the bellows (Fig. 2.6b,c). The tip of

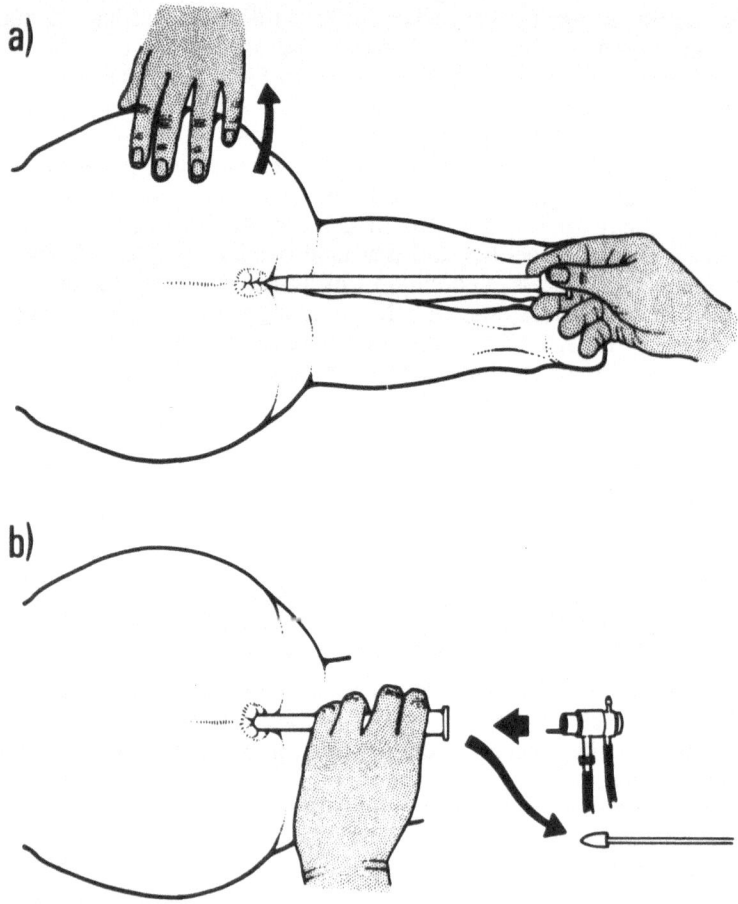

Fig. 2.6a–c. Rigid sigmoidoscopy.

c)

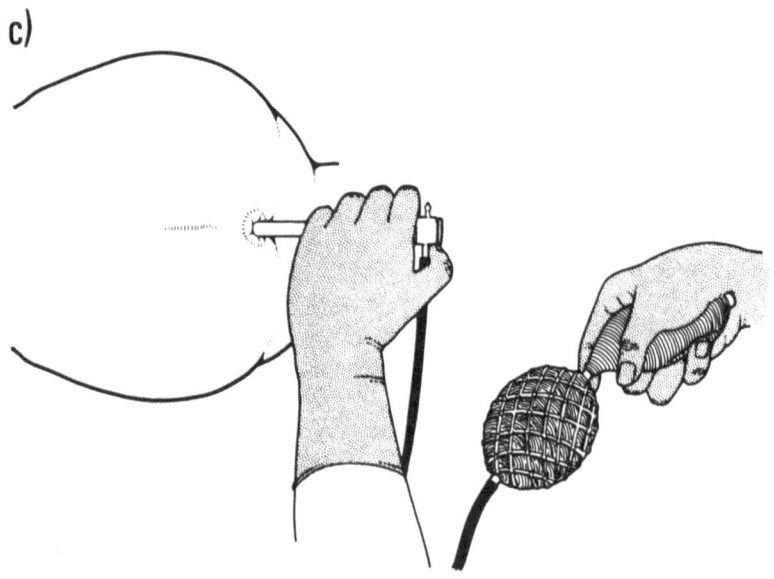

the instrument is angled backwards along the line of the sacral curve and advanced past the valves of Houston to the rectosigmoid junction, which lies at about 15 cm in the adult (Fig. 2.7). It is convenient for the examiner to sit down at this point since the rectum follows an anterior and leftwards path. Passing the rectosigmoid junction can be uncomfortable and should be done gently without forcing. Once the junction has been passed the instrument usually advances without difficulty up to the hilt. At about 18–20 cm the pulsations of the left iliac artery may be seen on the posterior medial wall.

A detailed examination of the mucosa is made on withdrawing the instrument, the tip of the sigmoidoscope being rotated in a spiral manner to cover all stretches of the mucosa including the areas just above the valves of Houston, where lesions (particularly adenomas) may be hidden.

The entire rectum can be seen in almost all cases and the success rate in passing the rectosigmoid junction is about 75%, being significantly higher in males (85%) than females (50%). The normal mucosa is smooth and sandy pink with a vascular pattern due to submucosal vessels that is seen in all areas; it does not bleed when touched by the instrument.

The distance to which the instrument has been passed should be recorded in centimetres from the anal verge after noting the calibration mark on the instrument that is level with the anal orifice when the instrument has been passed to its greatest extent.

The two golden rules of rigid sigmoidoscopy are to insufflate as little air as possible, and never to advance blindly or against resistance. The bowel can be perforated directly by the instrument or on taking a biopsy. The instrument should never be advanced if the patient complains of increasing pain. Perforation is more likely when sigmoidoscopy is performed under anaesthesia. Haemorrhage may follow trauma of an ulcerating lesion or after taking a biopsy.

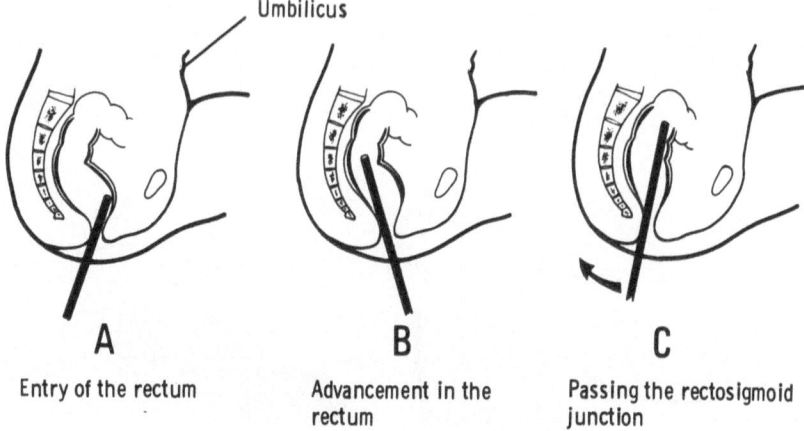

Fig. 2.7. Rigid sigmoidoscopy: direction taken by the instrument.

Although the paediatric sigmoidoscope is intended for use in babies and small children it can also be of great value in an adult with a painful anal lesion. The instrument has a diameter of 9 mm and can almost always be passed where the standard instrument might not be tolerated. Painful anal lesions may be associated with inflammatory bowel disease and it is essential to ensure the rectum is normal before treating the anal disease.

Abnormalities on Sigmoidoscopy

The presence of blood and/or pus in the lumen is a most significant sign since it indicates that disease is present somewhere in the bowel. If blood is present in the lumen a full investigation of the colon is obligatory. The site and extent of any mucosal lesion and its distance from the anal verge should be recorded on a diagram indicating the quadrants involved. With inflammation, the level of its upper limit (if visible) should be noted.

Abnormalities may be diffuse or localised. Diffuse mucosal involvement is a feature of inflammation, the initial abnormality being a loss of the normal vascular pattern due to oedema. This may occur with diarrhoea of any cause and is sometimes seen after the administration of an enema. More severe degrees of inflammation produce granularity, hyperaemia of the mucosa, contact bleeding, ulceration and inflammatory polyps. There are two morphological types of granularity. Fine granularity occurs in acute inflammation without fibrosis and appears as a regular pattern of minute elevations diffusely spread over the mucosa. It is due to mucosal oedema, which elevates the epithelium at all points except at the relatively fixed openings of the crypt glands. Coarse granularity occurs in chronic inflammation and appears as an irregular pattern of larger elevations of varying size (e.g. 1–3 mm). It is due to the combination of epithelial regeneration and repair with fibrosis after severe mucosal damage.

The commonest localised lesions are polyps. They vary in size from 1–2 mm to several centimetres and may be sessile or pedunculated, solitary or multiple. Sessile adenomas can be very extensive, for example occupying the circumference of the lumen over a distance of 10 cm or more. The number of polyps present, their sizes, distances from the anal verge and morphological appearances should be recorded.

Distal pedunculated polyps can be removed via the rigid sigmoidoscope by diathermy snare excision, but this should not be done until the rest of the bowel has been checked by an air contrast barium enema. If other polyps beyond the range of the instrument are found a colonoscopy is indicated to remove all lesions. If polyps are present in very large numbers, familial adenomatosis should be considered.

Carcinoma may be circumferential, producing a stricture, or confined to only part of the rectal wall. The typical raised everted edge and ulceration can be seen by sigmoidoscopy unless a stricture is too narrow for the instrument to pass. Hardness can sometimes be detected by moving the lesion with the tip of the sigmoidoscope. A solitary rectal ulcer may be impossible to distinguish from a carcinoma on appearances alone, and biopsy is required.

Other localised lesions seen on sigmoidoscopy include focal areas of Crohn's disease, the orifices of diverticula, the openings of fistula tracks, areas of trauma and previous anastomoses. A stricture may be caused by carcinoma, Crohn's disease, trauma, ischaemic bowel disease or radiation damage and very rarely by infections such as tuberculosis and lymphogranuloma venereum.

Proctoscopy

The anal canal is best examined with the proctoscope. This examination should be carried out after rigid sigmoidoscopy since treatment of haemorrhoids by injection, rubber band ligation, infrared coagulation or cryotherapy is most convenient at the end of the anorectal examination. Where flexible sigmoidoscopy is to be performed, proctoscopy should be deferred for the same reason. The standard proctoscope gives a circumferential view of the anal canal, but if a particular sector needs to be examined in detail the Graeme Anderson instrument affords a side view which is particularly useful for looking for the internal opening of a fistula-in-ano.

Technique (Fig. 2.8)

With the patient in the left lateral position the lubricated instrument is inserted in the direction of the umbilicus and the obturator is removed once the anorectal junction has been passed.

The anal canal is examined as the instrument is slowly withdrawn. The rectal mucosa begins to close the lumen at the level of the anorectal junction, below which the three bulges of the normal anal cushions at 3, 7 and 11 o'clock come into view. The dentate line is then recognised as a circumferential line of

serrations consisting of alternating anal valves and papillae which gives way to
the hairless skin of the anoderm below. Proctoscopy should be repeated while the
patient is asked to strain.

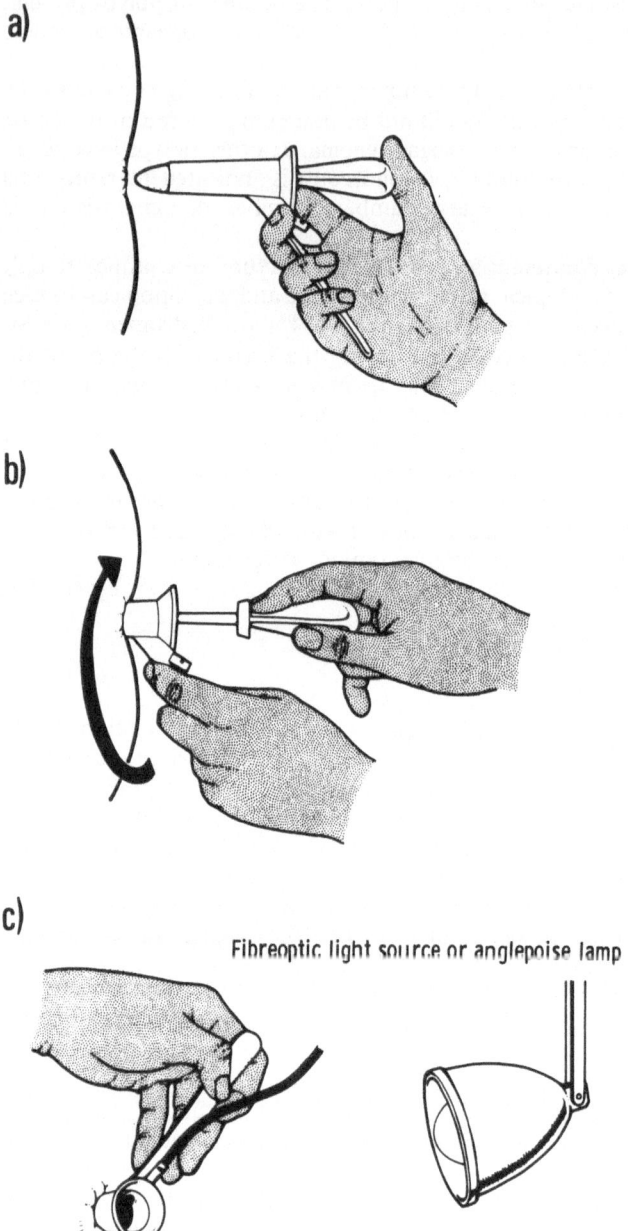

Fibreoptic light source or anglepoise lamp

Fig. 2.8a–c. Proctoscopy.

Abnormalities on Proctoscopy

Swellings, masses, ulcers, fissures, internal openings of fistulas and squamous metaplasia of the mucous membrane may all be seen. Haemorrhoids appear as swellings at the site of the normal anal cushions which often descend into the instrument particularly on straining. In most cases there are three located at the primary positions of 3, 7 and 11 o'clock, but they may also occur at intermediate sites. Squamous metaplasia is a histological term corresponding clinically to a whitened thickening of an area of mucous epithelium. It indicates frequent prolapse to the exterior and is found most commonly on the surface of a prolapsing haemorrhoid. Rectal mucosal prolapse is another common condition seen on proctoscopy. A fold of mucosa lying above the anorectal ring descends into the lumen of the instrument on straining. It occurs most often anteriorly but can involve the whole circumference of the bowel.

Ulceration may be seen in Crohn's disease and anal carcinoma. In cases of chronic fissure the apex of the nearest papilla of the dentate line may be hypertrophied. A hypertrophied anal papilla may also occur in the absence of any other anal disease as a so-called fibrous anal polyp.

Flexible Sigmoidoscopy

The flexible sigmoidoscope is 60 cm long and is potentially able, therefore, to reach at least to the splenic flexure. The immediate diagnosis of lesions too proximal for detection by the rigid sigmoidoscope can be a great advantage, especially if there is likely to be a delay between the first consultation and the barium enema examination. It must be remembered, however, that like rigid sigmoidoscopy, flexible sigmoidoscopy does not examine the large bowel fully and if negative must be followed by further investigation if colonic disease is suspected.

It has been shown that about four times the number of neoplasms, benign and malignant, are discovered by flexible compared with rigid sigmoidoscopy. This is particularly valuable in diagnosing carcinomas in the distal sigmoid colon which may occasionally be missed by rigid sigmoidoscopy and barium enema examination.

Indications

With an experienced operator flexible sigmoidoscopy takes about 5–10 minutes to perform. While it may not be logistically possible to examine all new patients, there are two strong indications for the examination: first where symptoms suggest a neoplasm but rigid sigmoidoscopy is negative, and secondly in cases of proctitis where the proximal extent of the inflammation cannot be determined by rigid sigmoidoscopy. It is also desirable that patients with an increased risk of having a carcinoma should be examined, including those with a previous history of adenoma or carcinoma, and with a family history of large bowel cancer.

Flexible sigmoidoscopy is also useful in cases where the barium enema has not produced a satisfactory examination of the sigmoid colon, particularly if symptoms suggest a colonic lesion. Some, including the authors, would maintain that the examination is indicated in all new patients over the age of forty.

Technique (Fig. 2.9)

The examination is carried out without sedation and the patient prepared with two disposable phosphate enemas. This will produce a clean bowel up to the splenic flexure in about 80% of cases. The patient lies in the left lateral position with only slight flexion of the hips and without the buttocks overhanging the edge of the couch as is necessary with rigid sigmoidoscopy. The instrument is lubricated and held in the left hand with its tip at the anus. The right index finger is inserted into the anus and the instrument is passed gently into the rectum as the finger is withdrawn (Fig. 2.9a).

The technique of advancing the instrument is similar to that of colonoscopy and the difficulties in passing flexures and traversing the sigmoid colon are equivalent. For a detailed description the reader is referred to standard textbooks on endoscopy, and the beginner is strongly advised to obtain practical instruction from a trained endoscopist. The suction and air buttons and the drive-wheels which control angulation of the tip are operated by the left hand. The shaft is held in the right hand which is responsible for inserting, withdrawing or rotating the instrument (Fig. 2.9b). The lumen should be kept in view at all times and this is achieved by a combination of angulation of the tip and rotation of the shaft. If the lumen disappears, the instrument should be withdrawn until it is seen once more; advancement can then be resumed. The introduction of air should be just

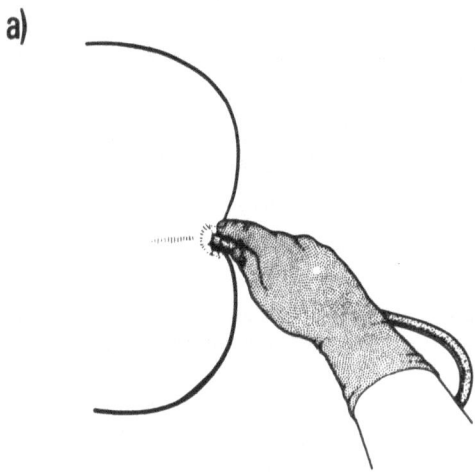

a)

Fig. 2.9a, b. Flexible sigmoidoscopy.

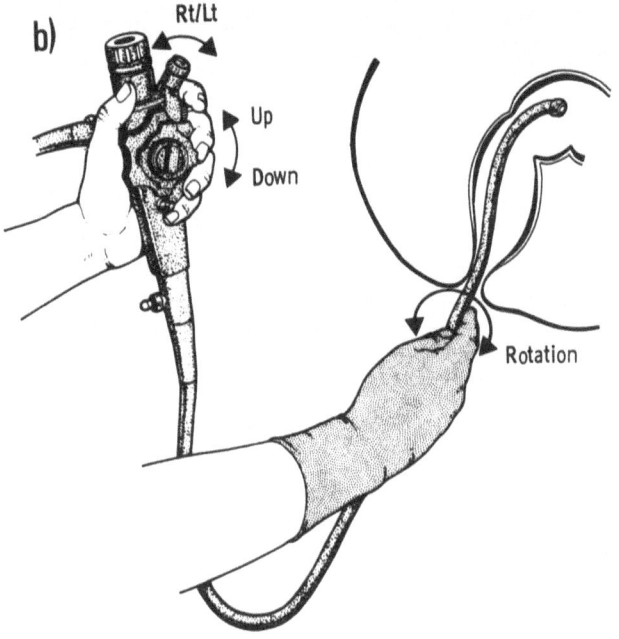

sufficient to obtain an adequate luminal view; distension of the bowel by air is a common cause of discomfort which may persist for several hours after the examination. Continued introduction of the instrument without advancement of the field of vision indicates that the bowel is being stretched, usually with the formation of a loop of sigmoid colon. This is another common cause of discomfort, and pushing under these circumstances must be avoided. When negotiating a sharp bend it may not be possible to see the lumen, but provided the mucosa moves across the field of vision as the instrument is gently advanced ('slide by') there is no danger of damaging the bowel. The instrument is inserted as far as possible and then as it is slowly withdrawn a careful search for abnormalities is made. Care should be taken to look for lesions behind folds and to avoid allowing the bowel to recoil proximally too rapidly for adequate inspection.

Without fluoroscopic screening, estimations of the anatomical extent of bowel examined are unreliable. On visual signs alone, however, the rectosigmoid junction can be identified and the sigmoid-descending junction frequently recognised as a flexure at about 35–45 cm. A rough guide to the extent of bowel examined is given by the calibration reading on the shaft that is level with the anal verge when the instrument is withdrawn. Average distances of rigid versus flexible sigmoidoscopy of 15–20 cm and 45–55 cm have been reported.

As with rigid sigmoidoscopy, the instrument should not be advanced if pain or resistance is encountered. Serious complications of flexible sigmoidoscopy are rare, but at least two cases of perforation, among several thousand examinations performed, have been reported. There appears to be little difference in discomfort experienced during rigid and flexible sigmoidoscopy in spite of the greater distance covered by the latter.

Biopsy Techniques

A mucosal biopsy can be performed either via the rigid sigmoidoscope or during colonoscopy or flexible sigmoidoscopy. The aim is to obtain a specimen, without complication, of adequate size for histopathological examination. A biopsy should not be carried out in patients with clotting disorders, including those taking anticoagulants or cytotoxic drugs or those with liver or renal disease.

Rigid Sigmoidoscopy (Fig. 2.10)

Large-cusp biopsy forceps produce satisfactory specimens but the site should be selected with some care when, as in diffuse inflammation, a choice is available. It is safer to take a specimen from the extraperitoneal part of the rectum, that is on the posterior or lateral walls below about 8–10 cm from the anal verge. The window attachment of the sigmoidoscope is removed and the forceps are introduced down the shaft. A generous portion of mucosa is grasped, the instrument rotated several times with the jaws closed while exerting gentle traction, and the specimen is detached. Rotation reduces the chance of bleeding, presumably by causing spasm of the submucosal vessels.

The biopsy specimen should be correctly orientated before it is fixed. Histological interpretation of a twisted or curled-up specimen is often difficult and it is the clinician's job to flatten it before fixation. The specimen is removed from the jaws of the forceps by a fine needle and laid out mucosa uppermost as a lamina on a small piece of ground glass. This is then gently placed in a pot containing formal mercury (mercuric chloride 70 g, commercial formalin 350 ml, water 2000 ml). If this is done carefully, the specimen stays on the glass. Formal mercury gives a more rapid fixation than formal saline.

Alternatively, the suction biopsy apparatus may be used. This employs the same principle as the Crosby capsule, drawing into a side hole in the instrument a tongue of mucosa which is then amputated by a guillotine knife operated by the examiner. This method has the advantages that larger specimens are obtained, orientation is easier and crush artefacts are avoided. However, it may cause artefactual congestion and is more likely to be followed by bleeding. It is only applicable where there is a diffuse lesion.

Complications include perforation and bleeding, and a biopsy should never be performed without inspecting the site afterwards. Some oozing is usual but occasionally a small vessel bleeding vigorously is seen. This is almost always controlled by local pressure from a swab held in the biopsy forceps, especially if the swab is soaked in a solution of topical adrenaline (1:1000). The patient should be re-examined 15 minutes or so later to check that the bleeding has not started

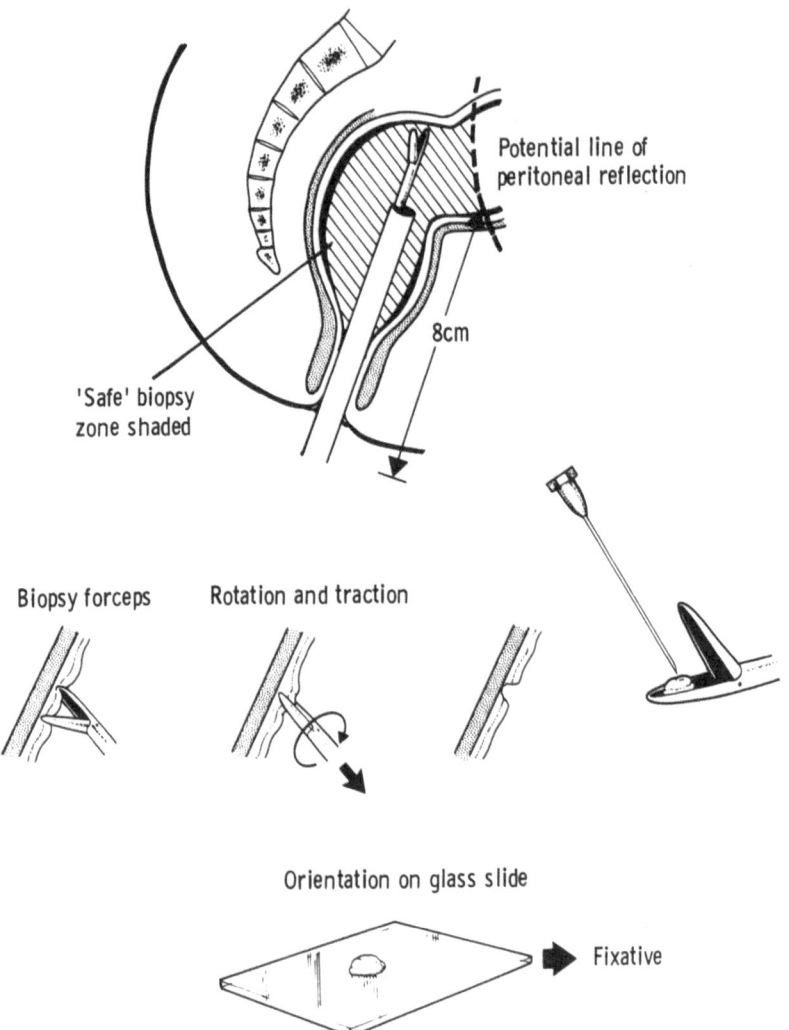

Fig. 2.10. Rectal biopsy through a rigid sigmoidoscope.

again. A barium enema examination might force a perforation at the biopsy site or worsen the consequences of an established perforation, so should not be performed within 10 days of a biopsy.

Flexible Endoscopy

The size of the specimen obtained using a flexible sigmoidoscope or colonoscope is much smaller and it is therefore not possible to orientate it as it is with a specimen obtained by rigid sigmoidoscopy. Specimens can, however, be obtained from different sites along the large bowel, enabling the extent and distribution of inflammatory bowel disease to be determined and increasing the chance of detecting severe dysplasia. Small polyps of 5 mm or less can be partially biopsied and the remainder completely destroyed by employing the hot biopsy technique. The polyp is grasped by the forceps and pulled away from the bowel wall into the lumen thereby creating a narrow stalk. Passage of a diathermy current across the polyp coagulates the stalk and the intact polyp is removed for examination. Larger pedunculated polyps and sessile polyps up to about 2.5 cm across can be removed as excision biopsy specimens by diathermy snare polypectomy, but both this and the hot biopsy technique are special procedures only to be carried out by trained colonoscopists. Bleeding and perforation occasionally occur.

Documentation

It is most important to record the sites from which biopsy specimens have been taken. With rigid sigmoidoscopy the distance from the anal verge and the circumferential quadrant should be recorded. It is more difficult with flexible endoscopy to be certain as to the precise location of a biopsy site, but with radiological screening the position of the instrument can be estimated with reasonable accuracy. If, as with flexible sigmoidoscopy, radiological screening is usually not available, the position can be roughly gauged by its relation to such landmarks as the rectosigmoid and the sigmoid–descending junctions.

Multiple biopsy specimens must be individually identified and placed in separately labelled pots. An alphabetical code is convenient, with the sites marked on a diagram in the notes.

Further Reading

Bohlman TW, Katon RM, Lipshutz GR, McCool MF, Smith FW, Melnyk CS (1977) Fibreoptic pansigmoidoscopy: An evaluation and comparison with rigid sigmoidoscopy. Gastroenterology 72: 644–649

Leicester RJ, Nicholls RJ, Pollett WG, Hawley PR (1982) Flexible sigmoidoscopy as an outpatient procedure. Lancet I: 34–35

Nicholls RJ (1984) The management of anorectal cases. In: Kyle J (ed) Pye's surgical handicraft. J Wright, Bristol, pp 438–460

Pugliese V, Bruzzi P, Aste H (1982) Left-sided colonoscopy in screening programs. What preparation? Endoscopy 14: 85–88

Sandler RS, Varma V, Herbst CA, Montana GS, Rudnick SA, Fowler WC (1982) Use of the flexible sigmoidoscope in women with previous pelvic irradiation. Gastrointest Endosc 28(4): 237–239

Vellacott KD, Amar SS, Hardcastle JD (1982) Comparison of rigid and flexible fibreoptic sigmoidoscopy with double contrast barium enemas. Br J Surg 69: 399–400

Winawer SJ, Leidner SD, Kurtz RC (1977) Flexible sigmoidoscopy compared to other diagnostic techniques in the detection of colorectal cancer and polyps. Gastrointest Endosc 23: 243–245

3 Special Investigations

Investigations must be justifiable and should not be requested before a full rectal examination that includes sigmoidoscopy. It is important to explain to the patient the reasons for and nature of further investigations to avoid confusion, anxiety and mistrust. The results of any investigations should always be considered in the light of clinical findings. A test may be repeated to clarify an equivocal result.

Sufficient information must be given on the request form. This should include a summary of symptoms, mention of previous diagnoses and operations, a statement of any relevant medication (for example antibiotics, vitamin B12) and a clinical diagnosis. Interpretation of difficult X-ray or histological appearances is often helped by discussion with the radiologist or pathologist.

Radiology

Plain X-ray Films

The radiologist will take a plain X-ray film of the abdomen routinely before carrying out a barium enema examination. It should, however, be requested before any further investigation if an acute abdominal condition is suspected or where abdominal distension is present.

Cases of peritonitis, perforation or strangulation are uncommon in the outpatient rectal clinic but subacute obstruction is found from time to time. Carcinoma or volvulus of the large bowel, ileocaecal or small intestinal Crohn's disease or adhesions and acute toxic dilatation may be present with distension. In cases of colitis toxic dilatation is considered present if the width of the colonic gas shadow is greater than 6 cm. If the condition is suspected from the clinical features, a sigmoidoscopy should be deferred until the plain abdominal X-ray film has been taken, since air introduced beforehand may confuse the radiological picture.

Faecal loading of the bowel may also be equally significant in patients with obstruction and in cases of constipation with or without megacolon. X-ray films of the spine and pelvis may reveal metastatic disease and a pelvic X-ray film is indicated if a presacral mass is present.

Intestinal Transit Rate

Estimation of intestinal transit rate is useful in the diagnosis of constipation. A known number of radio-opaque polyethylene shapes are given by mouth and a plain abdominal X-ray film is taken at 5 days. Intestinal transit is normal if 80% or more of the shapes have disappeared, whereas it is delayed if more than 20% are still present.

Barium Enema Examination

The chief indication for a barium enema examination is suspected colonic disease, but one should also be carried out in patients with a neoplasm already diagnosed by sigmoidoscopy in order to exclude a synchronous lesion and in proctitis if the proximal extent of the disease has not been determined by sigmoidoscopy. It is also indicated in the long-term follow-up of patients with neoplasms or ulcerative colitis where there is a risk of further neoplasia.

The examination is contraindicated in pregnancy or where there is a possibility of perforation, as in acute severe inflammatory bowel disease with colonic dilatation, acute diverticular disease with possible pericolic abscess and within 10 days of a sigmoidoscopic biopsy. The last restriction applies only to deep biopsy specimens taken with cusp biopsy forceps; those taken during fibre endoscopy do not penetrate beyond the submucosa and are therefore not liable to this hazard. The importance of a good bowel preparation should be emphasised to the patient. A low residue diet should be taken two days before and fluids only one day before the examination. A laxative such as castor oil (30 ml) or a senna preparation (e.g. X-Prep 70 ml) is given on the afternoon of the preceding day, and an hour before the examination two water enemas of total volume 2 litres are administered. Recently sodium picosulphate (Picolax) has been used instead of castor oil or senna. It is a strong stimulant laxative which when given in two spaced doses within the 24 hours preceding the barium enema gives an excellent bowel preparation in most cases.

Techniques

Two radiological techniques are in general use: the single contrast and the double air contrast barium enema. The latter gives such superior results, owing to its greater sensitivity in detecting mucosal abnormalities, that it should now be regarded as the method of choice.

In the single contrast barium enema, barium of low viscosity and density is introduced to fill the entire colon. The column of barium thus produced is then screened by fluoroscopy with the aim of detecting filling defects and other abnormalities in contour. Selected films are taken, the patient then evacuates the barium and further pictures are obtained. Mucosal detail is best seen in the post-evacuation films.

With the air contrast technique barium of a higher viscosity and density is used to coat the mucosa rather than to fill the lumen. Five hundred millilitres are introduced as far as the splenic flexure and after the majority has been evacuated by the patient, a litre of air is insufflated per rectum to push the barium coating the mucosa proximally to the caecum. During filling of the caecum the patient is placed in the prone position to avoid reflux of barium into the terminal ileum, since the ileocaecal valve then lies above the level of the barium at the caecal pole. A standard set of exposures with no fluoroscopic control is taken, to include prone, left lateral pelvic, right and left supine oblique, decubitus and erect views.

The strengths of the air contrast barium enema are the fine mucosal detail obtainable and the excellent views of the rectum and rectosigmoid junction that can be obtained. Lateral exposures demonstrate the post-rectal space as well as showing mucosal abnormalities of the rectum (Table 3.1).

Table 3.1. Barium enema: Advantages of double over single contrast technique

Greater diagnostic accuracy (carcinoma, polyps, inflammatory bowel disease)
Less barium to obscure views
Good views of rectum
No screening, thus less radiation and less radiologist time

While being guided by the radiologist's report, the clinician must look at all the films to check that the entire colon has been demonstrated and that overlapping of loops, particularly in the sigmoid colon, has not obscured parts of the bowel.

Instant Barium Enema

The instant barium enema is a modification of the full air contrast technique designed to determine the proximal extent of inflammation in patients with inflammatory bowel disease. No previous preparation is required since the bowel contains no formed faeces where the mucosa is inflamed. The examination takes only a few minutes and can therefore be carried out during the patient's first outpatient attendance.

An instant barium enema is indicated where diffuse rectal inflammation is found on sigmoidoscopy to extend beyond the range of examination. It is therefore chiefly applicable to cases of ulcerative colitis and is less suitable for patients with Crohn's disease of the colon since faeces may be present in normal segments between areas of disease. The examination is contraindicated in toxic megacolon. As with a fully prepared barium enema, it is also contraindicated after a sigmoidoscopic biopsy. If the radiologist is willing to perform an instant barium enema unforewarned, the patient can be sent directly to the X-ray department from the rectal clinic and asked to return immediately afterwards for a biopsy.

Oral Barium Studies

Barium Meal

A barium meal is designed to show the stomach and duodenum and gastro-oesophageal junction. Finer definition of the mucosa can be obtained using a double contrast technique following ingestion of an effervescent agent and water along with the barium.

Examination of the small bowel during a barium meal is unsatisfactory since there is poor coating of the mucosa by barium and too rapid a transit owing to the viscosity and density of the barium used. A clear distinction should therefore be made between a barium meal examination and a small bowel meal, and each examination requested separately.

Small Bowel Meal

The small bowel is best demonstrated by a small bowel meal in which dilute barium of a low viscosity is used. Unless the clinical picture is strongly suggestive of small bowel disease, a small bowel meal should be requested after a barium enema examination as barium is cleared more rapidly from the large than the small bowel.

After administration of the dilute barium the stomach and duodenum are screened and gastric emptying is encouraged by the administration of metoclopramide (Maxalon). Abdominal views are taken at 10-minute and then at 30-minute intervals until the caecum has been reached. The terminal ileum is screened and spot films are taken. Separation of small bowel loops is encouraged by direct abdominal pressure, either by palpation using a lead glove or by lying the patient on a balloon. Air contrast views of the terminal ileum can be obtained by insufflating air per rectum until reflux through the ileocaecal valve occurs. The small bowel meal will demonstrate strictures, mucosal irregularity, filling defects and diverticula.

Small Bowel Enema

In some centres a small bowel enema is used to obtain better definition of strictures by producing dilatation. Dilute barium is introduced directly to the proximal small bowel via an oral tube screened to lie in the fourth part of the duodenum. Two litres of dilute barium are infused over a 30-minute period followed by 600 ml of water to give a double contrast effect.

Intravenous Urography

An intravenous urogram may be indicated in patients with urinary symptoms or where bowel disease (for example diverticular disease, Crohn's disease or carcinoma) may be affecting the ureters or bladder.

Ultrasonography

The resolution of ultrasonography has improved considerably in recent years and modern machines can identify localised lesions down to 1.0 cm in diameter. Ultrasonography is useful in the detection of metastases, gallstones and intra-abdominal abscesses. Pelvic abscesses are less well defined owing to sound reflections from surrounding bone. Ultrasonic-directed needle biopsy or aspiration of abscesses has become a safe and useful technique. The accuracy of ultrasonography depends considerably on the technique of the examiner.

Computerised Tomography (CT)

CT gives good picture quality and is not as dependent on the examiner as is ultrasonography, although it is more costly. It is useful in identifying masses and their relationship to other organs. Its greatest application is therefore in malignant disease. Examination of extensive pelvic tumours may indicate involvement of other structures and help the surgeon to assess operability or to plan the extent of resection. It is also useful in identifying liver metastases or areas of recurrent tumour.

Colonoscopy

Colonoscopy is the most accurate method of investigating the large bowel mucosa and has the advantage over barium enema that tissue can be obtained for histological examination. It is, however, more time-consuming and in about 20% of patients it is technically impossible to examine the entire colon owing to redundancy or flexures in the bowel or to stricture formation. There is no indication for diagnostic colonoscopy if the barium enema examination is satisfactory and adequate for a clinical decision.

Indications

Colonoscopy is indicated where the results of the barium enema examination are equivocal or where symptoms remain unexplained after a normal barium enema. The accuracies of colonoscopy and barium enema examination in the right side of the colon are similar, but colonoscopy is superior in the left side, particularly in the sigmoid colon. Polyps and carcinomas in this part of the bowel may be missed on barium enema examination owing to the presence of diverticular disease or to overlapping of contrast-filled loops. A barium enema should be considered unsatisfactory if the caecum is not adequately distended or where a ring shadow suggesting a polyp cannot be distinguished from faecal residue or an air bubble. Vascular malformations, which are increasingly being recognised as a cause of intestinal bleeding, may be seen on colonoscopy but not on barium enema examination. The most useful applications of colonoscopy in the initial diagnosis are therefore to establish the cause of unexplained bleeding from the colon and to resolve equivocal radiological signs.

Colonoscopy may also be used to monitor disease and to detect the onset or recurrence of cancer in patients particularly at risk. It permits biopsy of lesions throughout the whole colon and the removal of polyps. Colonoscopic snare polypectomy is the treatment of choice for the majority of colonic polyps, about 95% being amenable to removal in this way. Contraindications for polypectomy include a polyp with a base wider than 2.5 cm or a polyp in which malignant change is strongly suspected from radiological signs. Small areas of angiodysplasia can be treated by diathermy fulguration at colonoscopy.

Technique

Full bowel preparation is essential for colonoscopy. There is a risk of explosion if electrosurgery is used after mannitol preparation since fermentation by gut bacteria may produce hydrogen. Preparation with dietary restriction, castor oil, senna (X-Prep) or sodium picosulphate (Picolax), and colonic washouts is satisfactory in most cases. (Carbon dioxide insufflation should be used during polypectomy to reduce the hazard of explosion.)

Sedation is usually necessary, a combination of diazepam (Valium) (5–20 mg intravenously) and pethidine (25–50 mg intravenously) being generally satisfactory. The patient should therefore come with a friend or relative to escort him home after the examination and be advised not to drive or operate machinery during the following 24 hours.

The technique of passing and advancing the instrument, which is an extension to that required for flexible sigmoidoscopy, is described in standard textbooks on endoscopy.

Pathological Tests

Examination of Faeces

Microbiology

If faeces are to be collected for microscopic examination it is better to obtain stool from within the rectum at sigmoidoscopy than to ask the patient to produce a specimen, since the specimen is assured and contamination with urine is avoided. Collection of faeces for microbiological examination is indicated in all cases of diarrhoea, inflammatory bowel disease and pruritus ani, and whenever possible specimens should be taken before any specific treatment is started.

If amoebiasis is suspected the stool should be examined within 3–4 hours and the microbiologist forewarned. Otherwise the specimen will remain in a satisfactory condition for culture and other tests for over 24 hours. It is not necessary to mix the stool with a transport medium or other solution, and specimens can conveniently be kept in a sterile leak-proof container overnight in a refrigerator at 4 °C if an urgent examination is not required.

The microbiologist should be informed of the symptoms and suspected diagnosis and it is important to state whether the patient is receiving anti-bacterial drugs, since they can markedly change bacterial morphology and impede or prevent growth. The microbiologist should also be told if the clinician suspects the presence of *Campylobacter* or *Clostridium difficile*, as these organisms are difficult to grow and require special conditions.

The stool sample is examined by direct microscopy and then cultured under aerobic and anaerobic conditions. Microscopy will identify most parasites while bacteria can only specifically be identified by culture and further tests such as fermentation reactions. Identification of viruses requires other specialised techniques. Most pathogens can be identified within 48 hours.

A brief list of organisms normally present in faeces and some important pathogens is given in Table 3.2.

Blood

There is little indication for examination of the faeces for blood in patients attending hospital since bleeding lesions should be identified by other investigation. However, testing for occult blood may have a place in the follow-up of patients who have already been treated for neoplasms as the presence of metachronous lesions may be detected in some cases. Its main role, however, is in the screening of non-hospital populations for large bowel cancer.

The test most commonly used is based on a reaction of the vegetable gum guaiac, which turns blue when oxidised. Haematin has a pseudoperoxidase action and splits the substrate hydrogen peroxide to produce molecular oxygen which reacts with guaiac. Commercial preparations which are available in kits suitable

Table 3.2. Some intestinal commensals and pathogens

1. Commensal bacteria
Enterobacter
Bacteroides
Clostridia
Lactobacillus
Streptococcus faecalis

2. Pathogens
Viruses
Rotavirus
Enterovirus
  Coxsackie A,B
  Polio
  Echovirus
Adenovirus
Unclassified small round virus
  Norwalk-like
  Ditchling-like

Bacteria
Enterobacter
  (certain *E. coli* serotypes)
Salmonella
Shigella
Vibrio cholera
Staphylococcus aureus
Yersinia

Protozoa
Entamoeba histolytica
Giardia lamblia
Trypanosoma cruzi

Metazoa
Nematodes (round worms)
  Ascaris lumbricoides
  Ankylostoma duodenale
  (hook worm)
  Necator americanus
  (hook worm)
  Enterobius vermicularis
  (threadworm, pinworm)
  Trichuris trichuria
  (whipworm)
  Strongyloides stercorales
Cestodes (tapeworms)
  Taenia solium
  Taenia saginata
  Diphilobothrium latum
  Echinococcus
Trematodes (flukes)
  Schistosoma mansoni
  Schistosoma japonicum
  Schistosoma intercalatum

Yeasts
Candida albicans

for transport by post include Haemoccult (Eaton Laboratories) and Faecatest (Labsystems). To diminish the number of false positive results the sensitivity of the test has been reduced by impregnating the guaiac in filter paper. False positives still occur, however, and may be due to dietary factors including peroxidase (for example from certain vegetables) and blood (for example in red meat), aspirin and vitamin C ingestion and non-neoplastic bleeding lesions (for example haemorrhoids). False negative results are due to faecal blood concentrations being too low for detection, to bleeding from lesions being intermittent and to faecal sampling error. Despite these drawbacks, the guaiac test of occult blood testing is the best method of screening for large bowel cancer at present and will detect about one cancer and five adenomas per 1000 individuals tested, of whom 30–40 will have been occult blood positive. Recently a screening test for blood based on the reaction of an antibody to human haemoglobin has been introduced. It should be more specific and the sensitivity can be adjusted by dilution.

Examination of Pus and Exudates

If possible, pus should be collected and placed into a sterile bottle, but where there is insufficient volume a culture swab usually suffices. Rapid transfer is most desirable since many organisms die with desiccation or when deprived of special conditions.

Material for examination for gonococci should be collected from the rectum, cervical fornices and urethral orifice either by a loop or a swab and transferred directly into a suitable transport medium (e.g. Stewart's medium). The specimens should be sent to the laboratory directly since incubation should start as soon as possible. Exudate from a suspected syphilitic lesion is collected directly into a sterile capillary tube or Pasteur pipette and gloves should be worn during this procedure. The spirochaete is looked for using dark-ground illumination or phase-contrast microscopy.

Infection of the perianal skin by fungi (tricophytes, epidermophytes) is an uncommon but treatable cause of pruritus ani. The diagnosis is made by seeing hyphae and spores on microscopical examination of scrapings taken from the skin. These should be obtained before the application of lubricant gel to the anus. A small scalpel blade held between finger and thumb is gently scraped several times over the skin and placed in a sterile pot (Fig. 3.1).

The ova of *Enterobius vermicularis* (threadworm) can be identified on microscopy. A length of transparent adhesive tape is applied to the perianal skin and then pressed onto a glass slide.

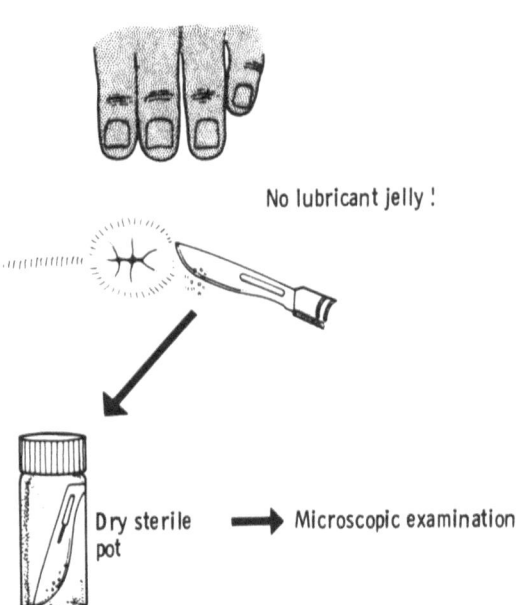

No lubricant jelly !

Dry sterile pot ⟶ Microscopic examination

Fig. 3.1. Taking a perianal skin scraping to identify fungal infections.

Examination of Blood

Estimation of haemoglobin, white cell count, erythrocyte sedimentation rate or electrolytes, or tests of liver function and for carcinoembryonic antigen may be indicated.

The presence of serum antibodies may be diagnostic of certain infections, especially if a rising titre can be demonstrated. In the early stages they may not be detectable and the rate of rise and fall of the antibody titre varies according to the disease.

Histology

The management of many diseases relies on the histological diagnosis. Biopsy during rigid or flexible sigmoidoscopy produces a sample of mucosa with some submucosa and is satisfactory in the majority of cases. In adult Hirschsprung's disease and in amyloid disease, however, a full thickness rectal biopsy is required, for which the patient should be admitted to hospital. A biopsy is contraindicated in patients taking anticoagulants or other drugs which may affect clotting.

In the absence of contraindications any undiagnosed mucosal lesion should be biopsied, including focal lesions such as carcinoma, polyps and solitary ulcer, and diffuse lesions such as those due to inflammatory bowel disease. As a general rule polyps should be removed by complete excision biopsy for two reasons: first if the lesion is an adenoma the pathologist may not have enough material to assess whether invasion of the muscularis mucosae indicating malignancy is present, and second the clinician may be unable subsequently to find the residual lesion to carry out complete removal.

Serial biopsies may be useful in gauging the response of inflammatory bowel disease to medical treatment. Patients with ulcerative colitis and to a lesser extent Crohn's disease are at a greater risk of developing large bowel cancer and histological demonstration of severe mucosal dysplasia may indicate impending or established cancer in some part of the large bowel. Regular endoscopy with biopsy of patients with unoperated extensive colitis or after colectomy with ileorectal anastomosis may be an effective means of cancer prevention if severe dysplasia is used as an indication for surgery.

Neuromuscular Anorectal Function

Studies of the neuromuscular function of the pelvic floor and anal sphincter may help in the assessment of patients with incontinence, megarectum, megacolon, prolapse and other pelvic floor disorders. Intraluminal pressure in the rectum and anal canal can be measured (manometry)) and action potentials of the muscles can be recorded using a needle electrode (electromyography).

Manometry

Pressure is measured using a small balloon probe (5-10 mm diameter) mounted on a catheter connected via a three-way tap to a pressure transducer in an air-free water-filled system. Pressure changes are converted into electrical impulses which after amplification are recorded on moving paper with an adjustable time-base. The system must first be calibrated against a water manometer and the voltage gain on the amplifier adjusted to the expected pressure range. A perfused open-tipped tube can also be used as the probe but is less satisfactory as it tends to become blocked by faeces.

Anal Canal Pressure (Fig. 3.2)

The anal canal pressure both at rest and during voluntary contraction of the pelvic floor can be measured by this method and it is also possible by withdrawing the probe from the rectum to the outside to obtain a pressure profile of the anal canal and thus to determine the functional length.

Manometry is best carried out with the patient in the left lateral position. The probe is inserted through the anal canal into the rectum and rectal pressure recorded. It is then withdrawn 1 cm at a time, recording the pressure with the patient at rest and during maximal voluntary contraction of the pelvic floor at each point during withdrawal. Maximal voluntary contraction pressure is the rise above the resting pressure occurring during contraction. Values range in the normal population as follows:

Resting anal canal pressure   50-100 cm water
Voluntary contraction pressure 60-120 cm water
Anal canal length   3-4 cm

Resting pressure is maintained by the internal and external anal sphincters, 60%-80% being due to the former which is thought to be in a state of maximal contraction. Voluntary contraction pressure is due to contraction of the external sphincter and puborectalis muscle.

Rectosphincteric Reflex (Fig. 3.3)

In normal individuals distension of the rectum produces a reflex fall in anal canal pressure. To measure this a large balloon (100-200 mm diameter) is inserted into the rectum and the same balloon probe as used for anal manometry is placed in the anal canal. Both catheters emerging from the anus are fixed to the patient's thigh with adhesive tape. Anal canal pressure is continuously monitored and after obtaining a baseline recording, 50 ml of air are injected into the rectal balloon. A sudden fall in anal canal pressure occurs, followed by a spontaneous rise towards the baseline level after a few seconds. With repeated injections of air, recovery of anal pressure becomes gradually less with each increment in the volume of the rectal balloon, until finally none occurs.

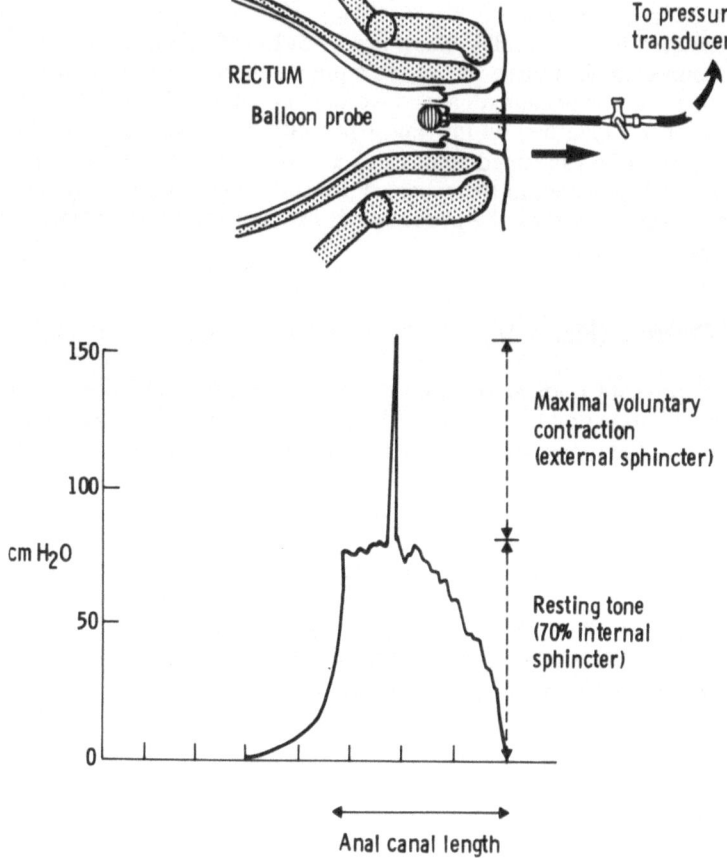

Fig. 3.2. Measurement of anal canal pressure using a balloon probe.

Abnormal Manometry

RESTING PRESSURE. Anal canal resting pressure falls immediately after proctoscopy but persistently low values may be due to trauma of the anal sphincter,
diffuse weakness of the pelvic floor musculature or a reflex reaction to rectal
distension. Trauma can result from lacerating injury or abnormal stretching, for
example by anal dilatation or in rectal prolapse where the prolapse itself acts as a
dilator. Weakness of the pelvic floor occurs in conditions causing denervation of
the levator ani and external sphincter. The reflex relaxation of the anal sphincter
found with faecal impaction of the rectum is caused by activation of the
rectosphincteric reflex.
    Increased resting anal canal pressure can be recorded in patients with anal
fissure and in some with haemorrhoids.

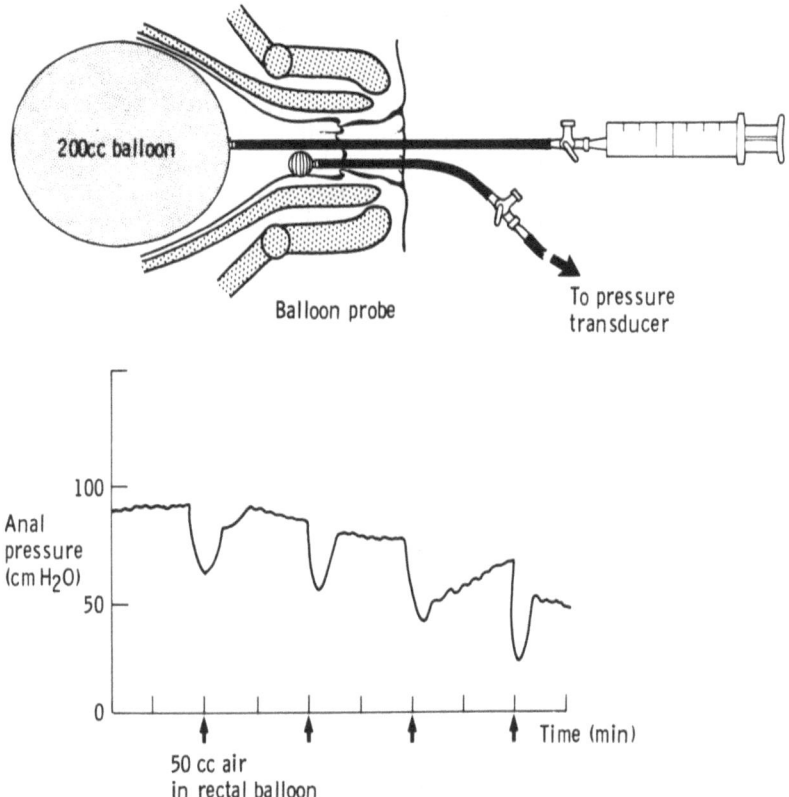

Fig. 3.3. Eliciting the rectosphincteric reflex: the normal response.

VOLUNTARY CONTRACTION. Reduced voluntary contraction is due to weakness of the external sphincter and puborectalis, which form part of the skeletal muscular component of the pelvic floor. This may follow direct lacerating trauma but more frequently is the result of diffuse denervation from demyelinating diseases, cauda equina lesions, or, more commonly, a neuropathy of the pudendal nerve and the levator ani branch of the fourth sacral nerve. Such neuropathy may occur as the result of traction injury, perhaps through perineal descent during childbirth or during prolonged and persistent straining at stool. A degree of denervation of the pelvic floor skeletal musculature occurs as part of the normal ageing process.

RECTOSPHINCTERIC REFLEX. The rectosphincteric reflex is absent in Hirschsprung's disease, in which no fall in anal pressure occurs during rectal distension. It is often absent in patients with abnormally low resting anal canal pressure, where perhaps any fall on rectal distension is too small to detect.

Electromyography

Electromyography can be useful in locating normally functioning pelvic floor muscle which has become disrupted by trauma or is distorted by congenital abnormality. In a specialised form of the technique it is possible to record activity from a single muscle fibre to give information on the degree of denervation of the pelvic floor. Its application to clinical problems is otherwise limited, but electromyography has been very valuable as a research tool in the study of the pathophysiology of incontinence and other pelvic floor disorders.

Further Reading

Ball AP (1982) Notes on infectious diseases. Churchill Livingstone, Edinburgh

Bartram CI, Kumar P (1980) Clinical radiology in gastroenterology. Blackwell Scientific, Oxford

Cotton PB, Williams CB (1980) Practical gastrointestinal endoscopy. Blackwell Scientific, Oxford

Doran J, Hardcastle JD (1982) Bleeding patterns in colorectal cancer, the effect of aspirin and the implications for faecal occult blood testing. Br J Surg 69: 711–713

Gnauk R (1982) Screeningtests nach Darmkrebs-erneuter Vergleich von Haemoccult mit hemo FEC und Rückblick auf 9 jahre klinische Erfahrung mit Haemoccult. Z Gastroenterol 20: 84–90

Hunt RH, Waye JD (1981) Colonoscopy. Chapman & Hall, London

Kuypers JD (1982) Anal manometry: Its applications and indications. Neth J Surg 34: 153–158

St John DJB, Caligiore P, Macrae FA (1981) Colorectal cancer screening. Med J Aust 2(8): 387–388

Taylor E, Phillips I (1980) Assessment of transport and isolation methods for gonococci. Br J Vener Dis 56: 390–393

Welin S, Welin G (1976) The double contrast examination of the colon. Experiences with the Welin modification. Georg Thieme, Stuttgart

Winawer SJ (1982) Sensitivity and specificity of the fecal occult blood test for colorectal neoplasia. Gastroenterology 82: 986–991

Wunderlich M (1982) Physiology and pathophysiology of the anal sphincters. Int Surg 67: 291–298

4 Clinical Presentations

In practice patients attending a rectal clinic complain of a limited number of symptoms. In each case the diagnosis is made after analysis of the symptom, construction of a differential diagnosis, physical examination and special investigations.

Present Complaint

It is essential to establish the time of onset of a symptom and how it has evolved up to the moment of presentation. Patients often need to be guided in building up their story in order that the periodicity of symptoms, their frequency, the nature of exacerbating and relieving factors, associations with other symptoms and possible predisposing causes can become apparent. Certain symptoms, particularly disturbances of bowel habit, may go back to childhood.

The symptom itself must be defined. What the patient means by diarrhoea, constipation, discharge, incontinence and even pain may be different from the doctor's understanding of these terms. A history sheet speeds up the consultation and ensures that potentially important symptoms are not missed (Table 4.1). Details of menstruation and urological symptoms should be obtained.

Past Medical History

Previous anorectal disease, cancer or polyps, abdominal operations and radiotherapy may all be relevant. Often patients with anal disease have had

Table 4.1. History sheet

Name _____ Age _____	

Number _____ Occupation _____

Date _____
Presenting symptoms:

Time of first onset _____

Bleeding	First onset _____ Colour _____
	Mixed with stool Yes/No Frequency _____

Bowel habit   Bowel actions/24 hours   _____ Consistency _____

Difficulty in defaecation   Yes/No   Straining   Yes/No

Anal pain
            on defaecation   Yes/No

Anal swelling

Discharge	Watery	Prolapse	Reducible
	Mucoid		Irreducible
	Purulent		
	Faecal		

Pruritus   Yes/No

Incontinence   First onset _____ Quantity _____

Frequency _____

Abdominal pain   Yes/No

Weight loss	Past Medical History
Appetite	
Urinary symptoms	Family History
Menstruation	
Drug History	Social History
Obstetric History	

treatment in the past. General medical diseases may produce colorectal symptoms and cardiac and respiratory disease is important when considering surgery.

Drug History

Several drugs can affect the bowel (Table 4.2). Certain aperients may possibly damage the colon and a history of cathartic ingestion for many years may be significant. It is essential to know whether a patient is taking anticoagulants if a

Table 4.2. Common drugs affecting the bowel

Diarrhoea	Constipation	Bleeding
Aperients	Opiates	Anticoagulants
Antibiotics	Anticholinergics	Drugs causing marrow
Magnesium antacids	Ganglion blockers	depression; cytotoxics;
Digitalis	Antidepressants	immunosuppressants
	(MAO inhibitors;	
	some tricyclics)	
	Iron	
	Calcium, aluminium	
	antacids	

biopsy or surgical treatment is contemplated, and patients on oral contraceptives should be identified.

Family History

The incidence of cancer among first-degree relatives of patients with large bowel cancer is about three to four times greater than in families without a history of cancer and there may, furthermore, be an increased familial incidence of adenoma formation. Patients with a family history of neoplasia should therefore be considered to be at increased risk of developing neoplasms. Both ulcerative colitis and Crohn's disease are more common among close relatives. The Mendelian dominant inheritance of polyposis syndromes is well established and family genealogies must be taken to identify others at risk. A history of abdominal operations within a family, especially if a colostomy was performed, may be a clue to a positive family history of bowel disease.

Obstetric History

The past obstetric history may be significant in patients with faecal incontinence and other disorders of the pelvic floor. The number of births, the duration of labour, the use of forceps and whether or not perineal tears occurred should be ascertained.

Bleeding

Almost all diseases of the large bowel and anus can cause bleeding. Bleeding may be symptomatic or it may be occult, only coming to light clinically as anaemia or through screening programmes for colorectal disease. Symptomatic bleeding can be minor or major, the latter being defined as bleeding causing clinical evidence of hypovolaemia.

Differential Diagnosis

The list of causes of bleeding is long and is summarised in Table 4.3, which also shows the order of examination and investigation required to make a diagnosis.

Table 4.3. Causes of bleeding and their diagnosis

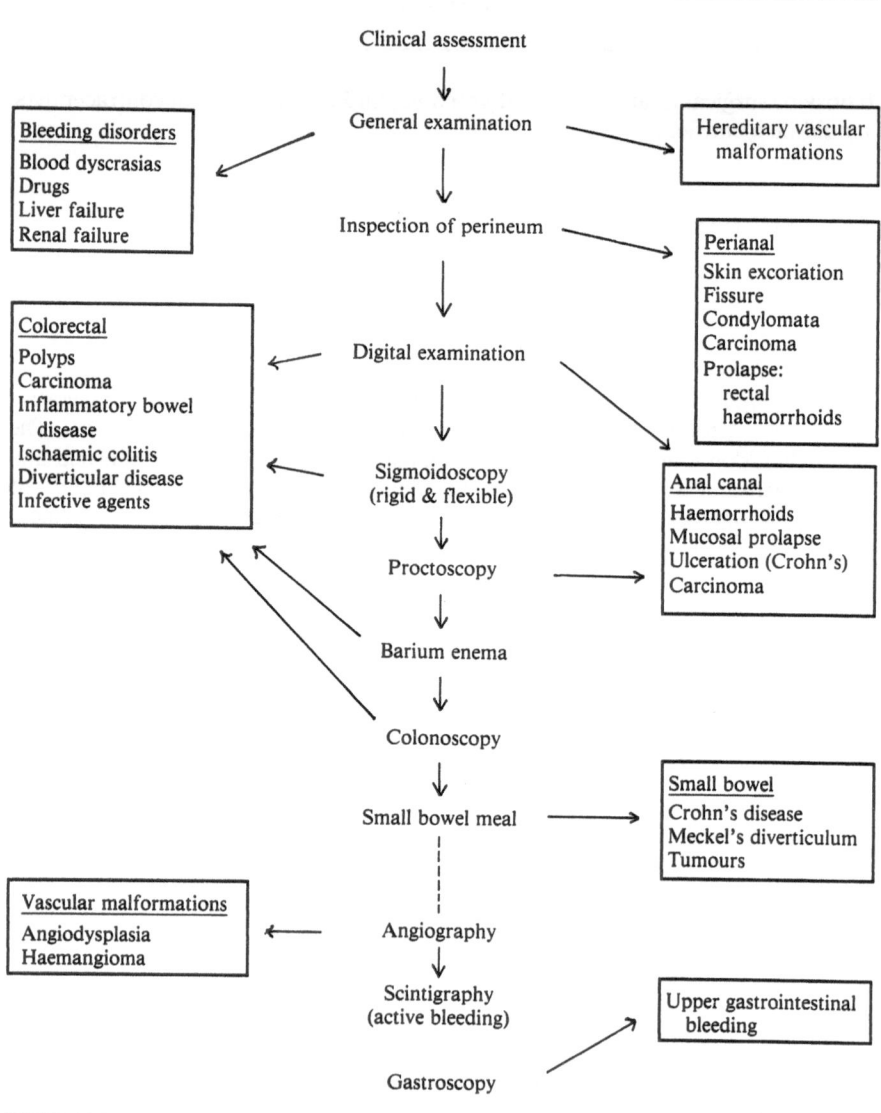

Minor Bleeding

Minor symptomatic bleeding is common and occurs in about 10% of the normal population aged between 25 and 65 years. Few of these individuals seek medical attention, presumably because the bleeding resolves and does not recur. The vast majority have haemorrhoids (80%) and fissure (15%), but a few (approximately 5%) have colorectal pathology.

The hospital referral pattern seems to be similar, with bleeding as the presenting symptom in 70% (308) of a series of 440 consecutive new patients attending the rectal clinic at St. Mark's Hospital, London. Of these, 79% were found to have an anal or perianal lesion, and 18% colorectal disease. In the remaining 3% no diagnosis was made (Fig. 4.1). As a reflection of this distribution, 85% of cases with bleeding were diagnosed by clinical examination, rigid sigmoidoscopy and proctoscopy, 10% by barium enema examination and/or flexible sigmoidoscopy and a further 2% by colonoscopy (Fig. 4.2). Most lesions can therefore be identified by relatively simple means.

Clinical Assessment

HISTORY. The length of history is often underestimated by the patient and careful questioning will double it in about 50% of cases. The colour of the blood, quantity, frequency and relationship to defaecation must be established.

LOCALISATION OF SOURCE. Bleeding from a site in the colon or upper rectum is suggested by the passage of dark red blood (like red wine, or plum-coloured), especially if the blood is mixed with the stool. Anal bleeding is typically bright in

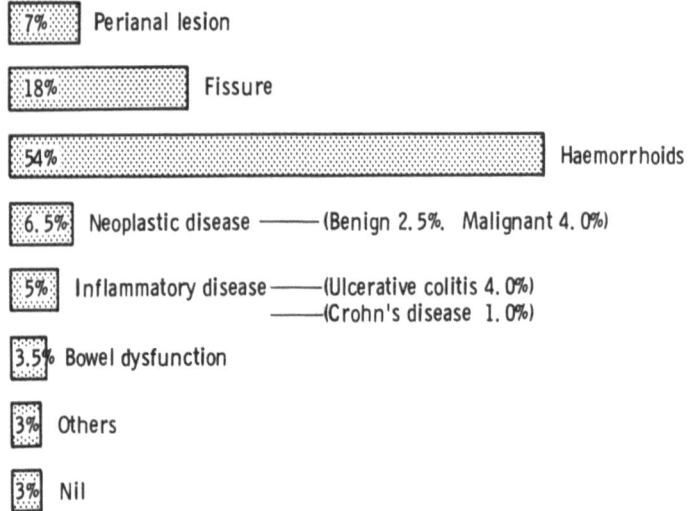

Fig. 4.1. Final diagnosis in 308 consecutive patients presenting with bleeding.

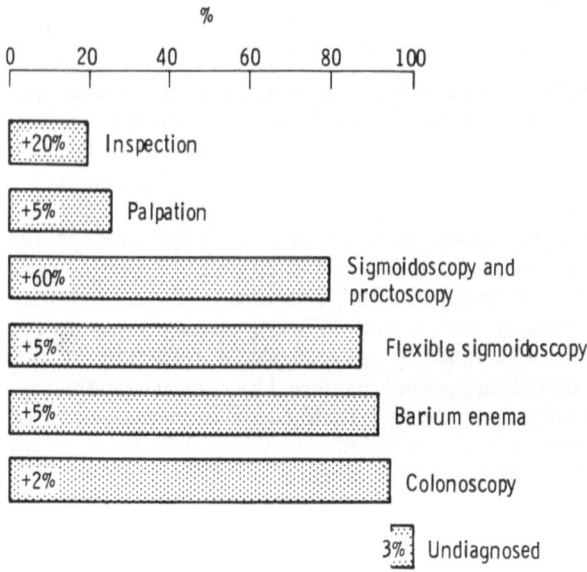

Fig. 4.2. Bleeding: efficacy of diagnostic methods.

colour (like blood from a cut finger), unmixed with the stool and often seen in the lavatory bowl. Blood on the toilet paper after wiping or seen as a stain on the underwear tends to be due to a lesion at the anal verge or in the perianal region.

These are, however, not hard and fast differences. Brisk bleeding from the colon or even the more proximal intestine may be bright and unmixed and dark bleeding may occur from an anal lesion, for example haemorrhoids, where blood has been retained in the lower rectum for some time before being passed.

OTHER SYMPTOMS. Alteration in bowel habit, abdominal pain and general symptoms, such as anorexia and weight loss, suggest disease in the large or small bowel as opposed to the anus. The passage of mucus occurs in both anal and more proximal disease.

Examination

Medical diseases causing bleeding are diagnosed on the general examination with appropriate investigations. As can be seen in Table 4.3 inspection of the perineum will identify many simple conditions. Every effort must be made to feel as much of the rectum as possible by digital examination. Special attention should be given to the posterior rectum just above the anorectal ring where it is often difficult to obtain a good view on sigmoidoscopy. Polyps, especially sessile adenomas, may be so soft as to be difficult to distinguish from normal mucosa and haemorrhoids cannot be diagnosed by digital examination. Besides diagnosis, digital examination enables an assessment of the extent and degree of invasion of polyps and carcinoma.

All patients must have rigid sigmoidoscopy. In 95% of cases the entire rectum can be seen and a biopsy or bacteriological swab of any lesion can be taken. Flexible sigmoidoscopy is highly desirable in patients in whom a colonic lesion is suspected from the history or in those at greater risk of having a neoplasm. The possible diagnoses are no different from those seen on rigid sigmoidoscopy but the yield of neoplasms is about four times greater. Diverticula, which are only occasionally seen on rigid sigmoidoscopy, are commonly found when the sigmoid colon is visualised.

The diagnosis of haemorrhoids is made on proctoscopy, which may show other anal canal lesions that can cause bleeding, such as ulceration and also prolapse of the lower rectal mucosa.

Investigation

A barium enema examination must be requested when a diagnosis has not been made by sigmoidoscopy. It is also required in inflammatory bowel disease to determine the extent of inflammation and, where a neoplasm has been identified, to exclude synchronous lesions. If in doubt it is safer to request a barium enema than not. A small bowel meal is indicated where examination of the large bowel is negative or where Crohn's disease is suspected or has already been diagnosed in the large bowel.

Colonoscopy is indicated if the barium enema examination is normal. Certain lesions, particularly mild inflammatory disease and angiodysplasia, may be identified. Colonoscopy can be expected to allow a diagnosis in around 50%–60% of patients with bleeding and a normal barium enema, and 10%–20% of these will be found to have a carcinoma. When directly compared, a barium enema is less sensitive than colonoscopy, and a barium enema examination showing only severe diverticular disease does not exclude carcinoma in that part of the bowel. Despite these disadvantages, barium enema remains the first investigation for total examination of the large bowel. In the hands of an experienced radiologist it is quick, easy to perform and provides a permanent record. However, attention to technique is important in minimising false negative examinations.

Colonoscopy itself is liable to false negatives: for example as many as 50% of patients who have an initial polypectomy for adenoma may be found to have further polyps on re-examination within a year, suggesting (particularly if the polyps are over 10 mm in diameter) that some are missed on the first examination.

Failure of colonoscopy to allow a diagnosis in patients with bleeding and a normal barium enema examination has been reported in up to 50% of cases. It is in this small group, representing about 2% of all patients with bleeding, that angiography may be helpful. The most common lesions found are angiodysplasia and other vascular malformations, but in about 25% of these patients the bleeding is ultimately discovered to have an upper gastrointestinal cause. Thus a gastroscopy should be carried out where a diagnosis has not been made after colonoscopy. There remains, however, a small number of patients in whom the cause of bleeding is not found.

Major Bleeding

Major bleeding from the lower gastrointestinal tract is much less common and
the patient often presents as an emergency. The relative incidence of diseases
causing it is different from the pattern associated with minor bleeding, with
diverticular disease and angiodysplasia together accounting for over 50% of
cases. Tumours, ulcerative colitis, Crohn's disease and ischaemic bowel disease
comprise 10%–15% of cases and rarer causes include Meckel's diverticulum,
radiation enteritis, solitary ulcer and haemorrhoids.

In the 1960s it began to be appreciated that bleeding from diverticular disease
was more likely to come from the right than the left colon, and with the
introduction of angiography it has been demonstrated that some of these cases
are due to angiodysplasia. The reported incidence of angiodysplasia is, however,
variable.

In patients with active bleeding radiolabelled red cell scintigraphy to localise
the site is now preferred to angiography.

Discharge

Patients often complain of a discharge or moisture in the perianal region which in
most cases is due to a pathological lesion, although poor anal hygiene is
responsible in some. Discharge may produce an offensive smell which is often the
main reason for presentation of the patient.

Differential Diagnosis (Table 4.4)

The nature of the discharge, the presence of other symptoms and the site of
origin should be determined.

Clinical Assessment

History

Discharge may be watery, mucoid, purulent or faecal. A faecal discharge does
not necessarily mean incontinence for some faecal staining of a watery or mucous
discharge may be present if anal hygiene is difficult to maintain. A purulent
discharge limits the diagnosis to septic lesions: only rarely does inflammatory
bowel disease produce pus.

The association of discharge with other symptoms such as pruritus, bleeding,
pain and prolapse is helpful in diagnosis (Table 4.5). Pruritus may simply be a
consequence of the discharge, which per se damages and and irritates the perianal
skin.

Table 4.4. Anal discharge: Causes

Type of discharge	Site		
	Perianal	Anal	Colorectal
Watery/mucoid	Sweat/poor anal hygiene Skin excoriation Fissure Condylomata	Condylomata	—
	Carcinoma	Haemorrhoids Mucosal prolapse	Rectal prolapse Inflammatory bowel disease Solitary ulcer Adenoma Irritable bowel syndrome
Purulent	Fissure Abscess Fistula Hidradenitis Furuncle	Fistula Abscess	Inflammatory bowel disease
Faecal	Poor anal hygiene	Any cause of incontinence	

Table 4.5. Anal discharge: Association with other symptoms

Type of discharge	Pain	Pruritus	Blood	Prolapse
Watery/mucoid	Fissure	Fissure Other perianal lesions Poor anal hygiene	Fissure Haemorrhoids Colorectal lesion	Haemorrhoids Rectal prolapse Mucosal prolapse
Purulent	Fistula/abscess	Fistula/abscess		
Faecal		Poor anal hygiene Incontinence		

Examination and Investigation

Perianal and prolapsing lesions are identified on direct inspection and the remainder on full anorectal examination with investigation of the large bowel if necessary. Digital examination is particularly important in the diagnosis of fistula. In suspected cases of sexually transmitted disease or fungal infection, serological and microbiological tests should be requested.

Incontinence

Faecal incontinence is a most disabling symptom. It is frequently concealed by the patient out of shame and embarrassment. Sufferers are often reduced to a life confined to the house and they may be rejected by their family and friends.

Mechanisms of Continence

Continence depends on two factors: the consistency of the stool and the competence of the anal sphincter mechanism.

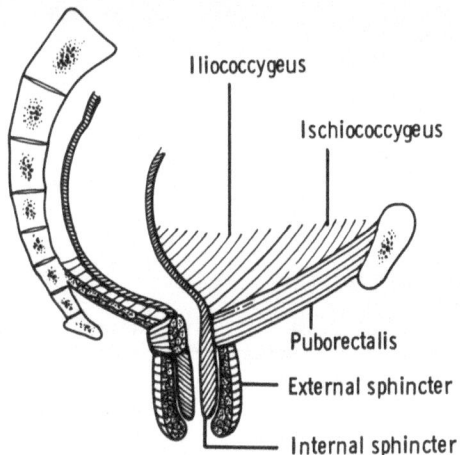

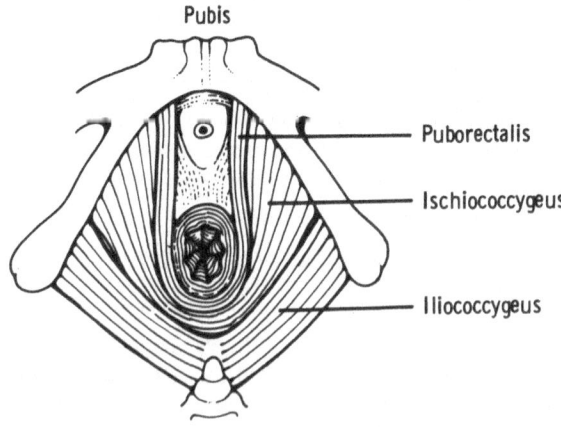

Fig. 4.3. Anatomy of the pelvic floor.

A sphincter which can hold formed stool may, particularly if weakened, fail to do so if the stool is liquid or where irritability of the rectum causes urgency. The competence of the anal sphincter mechanism is itself a function of two factors: namely the anorectal angle and closure of the anal canal, both of which are maintained by the pelvic floor musculature (Fig. 4.3). This musculature consists of a skeletal part and a visceral part. The skeletal part, which includes the levator ani, puborectalis and external sphincter, is one anatomical continuum which invests the gut tube. It is in a constant state of tonic activity even during sleep, maintained by muscle spindle stretch reflexes mediated through the extrapyramidal system. Tone is therefore increased in response to stretch caused by raised intra-abdominal pressure, e.g. during coughing. The visceral part is formed by the smooth muscle internal sphincter of the anal canal, which is in a state of maximal contraction at rest.

Anorectal Angle

The levator ani consists of the ischio- and ileococcygeus muscles which form a sheet across the pelvic outlet supporting the pelvic viscera. The puborectalis is a specialised part of the levator which passes immediately behind the gut tube as it perforates the pelvic floor and maintains the anorectal angle. Under normal circumstances this angle is about 90 degrees and the sling which can be felt posteriorly on digital examination defines the level of the anorectal junction (Fig. 4.4).

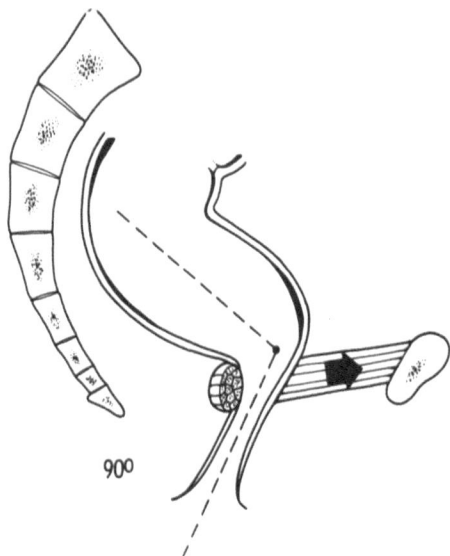

Fig. 4.4. The normal anorectal angle.

Anal Canal Closure

Closure of the anal canal is due to the combined action of the internal and external sphincters. Normal resting anal canal pressure lies between 60 and 100 cm of water, of which 60%–80% is maintained by the internal sphincter. The external sphincter thus contributes approximately 20%–40% to resting tone, but is exclusively responsible for the rise in pressure which occurs during voluntary contraction. This can attain values above resting pressure of 100 cm of water or more in normal individuals. Distension of the rectum causes a fall in anal canal pressure (the rectosphincteric reflex) the extent of which is related to the degree of rectal distension.

Differential Diagnosis

Diarrhoea is the commonest cause of incontinence and even in patients with a normal sphincter mechanism it may occur when the stool is liquid and there is urgency. Incontinence can therefore be a feature of any condition causing diarrhoea.

The anal sphincter mechanism may be deficient owing to muscular weakness. Denervation may occur in general neurological diseases such as disseminated sclerosis and following spinal injury that causes damage to the cauda equina. A patchy diffuse denervation of the levator is a normal part of ageing, the process accelerating after the age of 70 years; a similar diffuse type of denervation may also occur in younger patients in whom physiological and histocytochemical studies have demonstrated a lower motor neuropathy affecting the pelvic floor muscles. Complete rectal prolapse and pelvic floor neuropathy are frequently associated.

Incontinence may occur in cases of faecal impaction where distension of the rectum has produced reflex relaxation of the internal sphincter.

The sphincter mechanism may be disrupted locally by trauma, including lacerating injuries and surgical operations. Indeed anal fistula surgery is the commonest cause of traumatic incontinence.

Incontinence will occur where the anal sphincter is by-passed by virtue of a fistula from the rectum to the exterior above the level of the anorectal junction. Rectovaginal or extrarectal fistulas to the perineum may be congenital or acquired as the result of trauma, specific diseases (for example Crohn's disease or carcinoma) or following radiotherapy usually for carcinoma of the cervix.

The causes of incontinence and their diagnosis are summarised in Table 4.6.

Clinical Assessment

History

The history should first distinguish between discharge and faecal incontinence, since patients may confuse the two symptoms. The severity should then be

Table 4.6. Incontinence: Causes and diagnosis

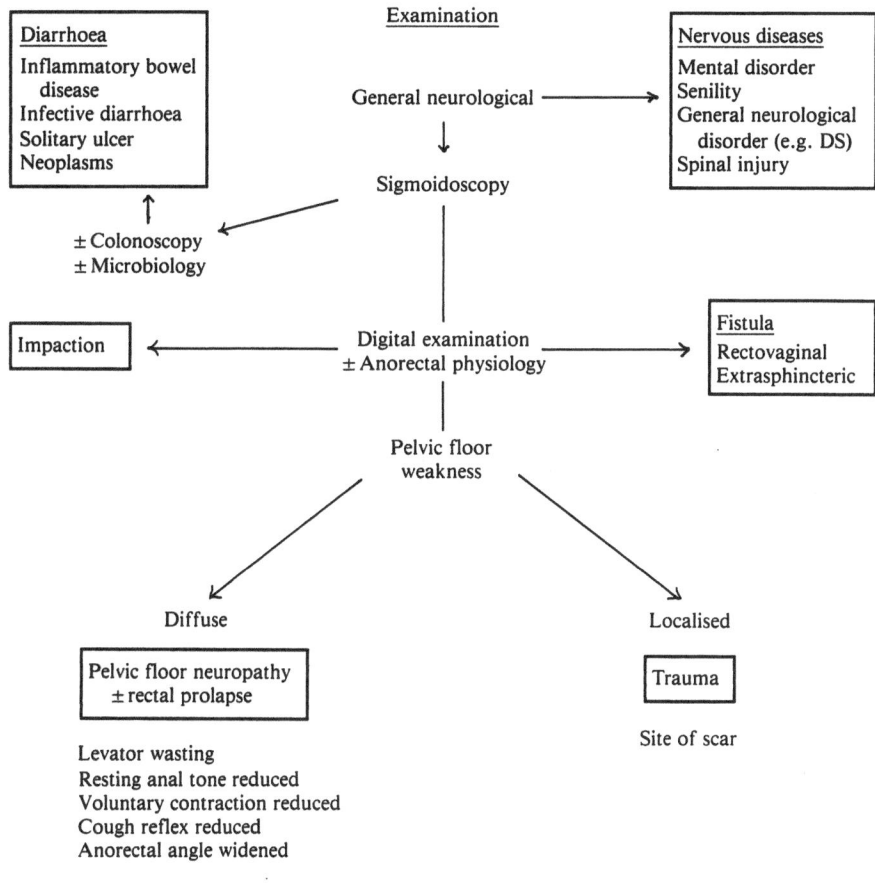

determined by an assessment of the frequency of incontinence and the amount of the faeces lost on each occasion. There is a great difference between the leakage of flatus or an occasional smear on the underclothing and the involuntary loss of a formed faecal bolus several times a day. The consistency of the stool—whether watery, porridge-like or formed—is also important and frequency and urgency of defaecation may indicate that some form of diarrhoea is the cause. A past history with particular reference to previous anal operations (especially for fistula), radiotherapy, and spinal or perineal trauma must be taken, as must a full obstetric history.

Examination

Signs of general neurological diseases and a cauda equina lesion should be looked for and an assessment of the mental state of the patient made.

Anorectal Examination

INSPECTION. Faecal soiling around the anus, any patulosity of the anal orifice, rectal or mucosal prolapse and perineal scarring are noted. Voluntary contraction of the perineum will give a useful impression of the power of skeletal muscle contraction, and is the most useful means of locating muscle after lacerating injury. On straining there may be abnormal perineal descent or prolapse, either mucosal or complete. A diagnosis of impaction is made on inspection and digital examination.

DIGITAL EXAMINATION. Palpation of the entire pelvic musculature is possible. At rest the muscle bulk of the levator ani can be estimated and the anorectal angle and resting anal canal tone assessed. The power of the puborectalis and external sphincter on voluntary contraction is estimated and the cough reflex assessed.

Digital examination will distinguish between patients with a diffuse generalised weakness of the pelvic floor (i.e. neuropathic) and those with a localised disruption of the anorectal ring (i.e. traumatic). In the former, anal canal resting tone and voluntary contraction are reduced or even absent, there is widening of the anorectal angle, reduction in bulk of the levator ani on both sides and a reduced or absent cough reflex. In the latter, muscle tone and contraction are likely to be normal but the sphincter is unable, owing to the injury, to achieve adequate anal canal closure. The essential physical sign to elicit in trauma is the site of scarring.

ANORECTAL PHYSIOLOGY. Manometry and electromyography have contributed greatly to understanding the pathophysiology of incontinence. However, from the practical point of view management is based more on clinical than physiological assessment. There is generally good correlation between them and the latter has the advantage of providing a permanent record and an objective means of assessing any improvement following surgery. In most patients with incontinence resting and voluntary contraction pressures are below the normal lower limits of 50 and 60 cm of water respectively. Maximal voluntary contraction pressure—which effectively assesses external sphincter power—is often very low or even absent in patients with pelvic floor neuropathy.

The practical value of electromyography in deciding on the type of operation is limited, but it may enable skeletal muscle to be identified in cases of trauma or congenital anomaly where the normal anatomical arrangement has been distorted. Single-fibre electromyography can identify denervation and give a quantitative estimate of its degree.

Pruritus Ani

Pruritus ani is a symptom not a disease and occurs in many conditions. Irritation or soreness should be distinguished from pain. The severity can be gauged from an assessment of the intensity and periodicity and whether normal activity such as sleep is disturbed.

Mechanisms

Pruritus can be caused through direct damage to the perianal skin by primary skin diseases or local perianal conditions, or it can be secondary to moisture or faecal soiling.

The perianal area is normally colonised by skin commensals but faecal organisms can be cultured from a perineal swab in a high proportion of patients with pruritus. Faecal bacteria produce metabolites some of which, for example neuramidases, are among the most powerful skin irritants known. Moisture through sweat or mucus causes maceration and excoriation of the skin and the irritation resulting from these factors sets up a vicious circle since the patient scratches to obtain relief but further damages the skin in doing so.

Any lesion which produces a discharge can therefore cause pruritus.

Differential Diagnosis (Table 4.7)

Generalised dermatoses account for about 5% of cases presenting to a rectal clinic and local perianal conditions for a further 30%–40%. Contact dermatitis, often due to local anaesthetic application, occurs in about 5% of patients. General medical diseases are rare causes of pruritus ani and the majority of cases are therefore due to secondary skin damage. It has recently been recognised that this last category contains a subgroup of patients in whom the only demonstrable abnormality is an exaggerated and prolonged reduction in anal canal resting tone on rectal distension which may lead to a minor degree of soiling. More often, however, poor anal hygiene is due to inadequate cleaning after defaecation. This may be difficult in hirsute or sweaty individuals or if skin tags or prolapsed haemorrhoids are present. Patients with diarrhoea often develop anal soreness. As with any symptom, in some patients no cause can be found.

Clinical Assessment

History

The presence or absence of the following symptoms should be established: skin irritation or eruptions elsewhere on the body, anal discharge whether mucus or

Table 4.7. Pruritus ani: Causes

Primary	
Generalised dermatoses	Eczema
	Psoriasis
	Lichen planus
	Allergic eruptions
Perianal disease	
Local lesion	Fissure
	Carcinoma
	Crohn's disease
Infection	Fungal
	Yeast
	Worms
	Sexually transmitted diseases
	(condylomata acuminata, chancre, herpes)
Contact dermatitis	Local anaesthetics
	Antibiotic ointment
Secondary	
Skin damage due to moisture and irritants	
Sweat	Poor anal hygiene
Mucus	Prolapse (rectal, haemorrhoids)
	Mucus overproduction
	(adenoma, carcinoma,
	solitary ulcer)
Pus	Fistula-in-ano
Faeces	Diarrhoea
	Incontinence
	Poor anal hygiene
General medical diseases	Diabetes mellitus
	Myeloproliferative disorders
	Obstructive jaundice
	Lymphoma
Idiopathic	

pus, faecal soiling, pain suggesting a fissure or fistula, prolapse, and diarrhoea. The patient should be asked about allergies and details of suppositories or local preparations used on the anal skin. Worm infestations often affect other members of the family. A history of anogenital contact may be relevant.

Examination and Investigation (Table 4.8)

General examination and appropriate investigations will exclude dermatoses and medical diseases. On inspection of the anus the following signs should be looked for: moisture and soiling, skin maceration and excoriation, a skin eruption, perianal lesions and prolapse. Faecal soiling can be detected by wiping the anus with a tissue which will stain brown. A lax anal orifice is an indication both of a weak sphincter and of possible prolapse. Digital examination, sigmoidoscopy and proctoscopy will identify cases of sphincter incompetence, fistula, haemorrhoids and mucus-producing rectal lesions.

Table 4.8. Pruritus ani: Diagnosis

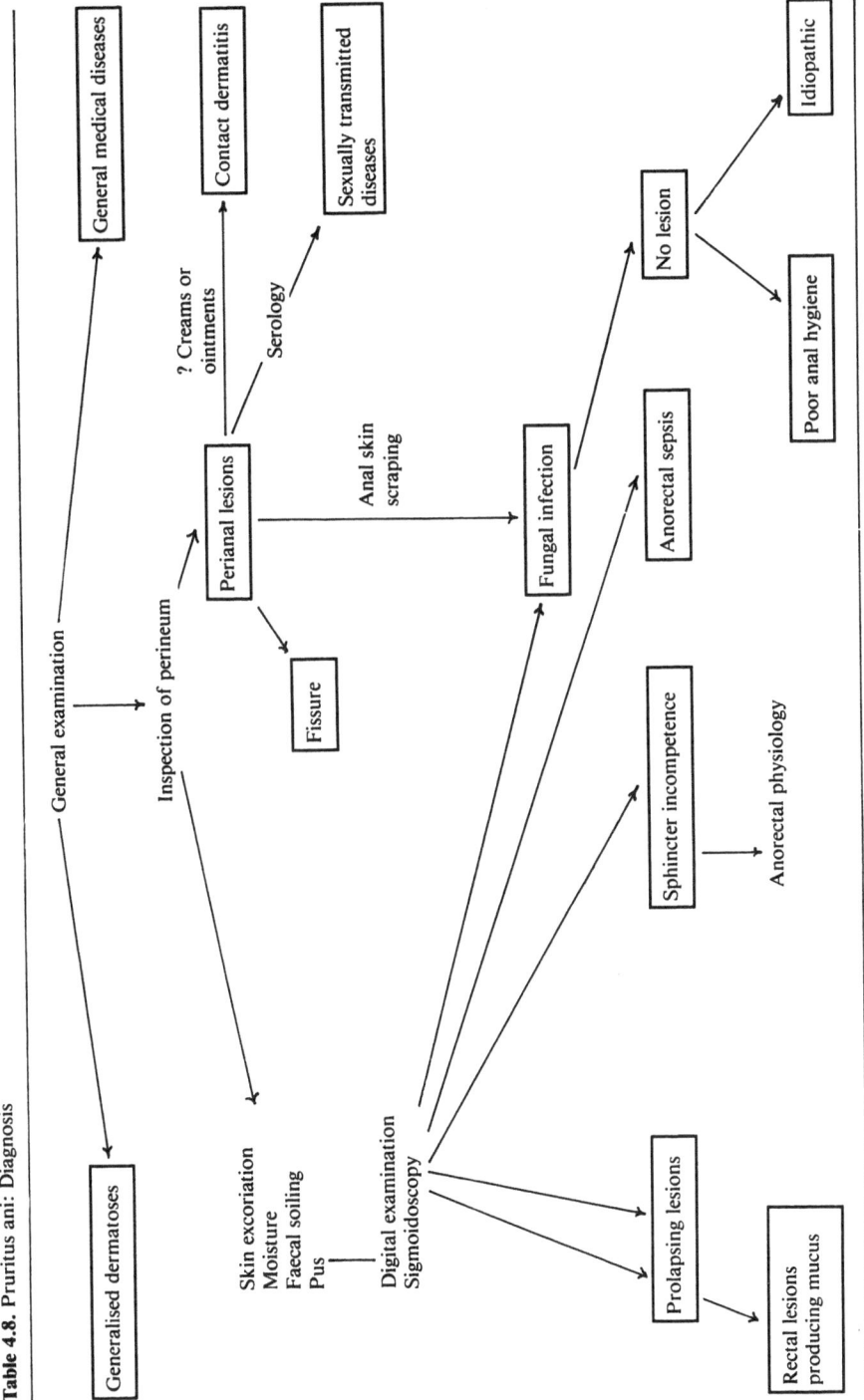

It is wise to take an anal skin scraping for microbiological examination for fungal infection in all cases and serological tests should be requested if sexually transmitted disease is suspected. Stool microbiology is indicated in cases of diarrhoea, a rectal lesion should be biopsied, and anorectal physiology studied in patients with sphincter incompetence. Worm infestation can be diagnosed by microscopic examination of a swab from the perianal skin to show ova.

Management

Management is a combination of general measures and treatment of any underlying cause.

General measures include the avoidance of trauma and attempts to maintain the anal region clean and dry. Local anaesthetic preparations and any other allergenic agent, e.g. soap, are proscribed. Trauma by scratching must be stopped and the patient is advised to use soft tissue for cleaning the anus after defaecation. Any faecal remnants are removed by moist tissue and the anus then carefully dried. Local preparations such as zinc borate starch dusting powder, magnesium carbol lotion and talcum powder help to keep the region dry. Steroid preparations are advised by some.

Perineal Pain

Differential Diagnosis (Table 4.9)

Perineal pain is a common presentation. It may be caused by conditions affecting the anus, rectum or other pelvic organs and failure to identify the site will lead to a wrong diagnosis and treatment.

Clinical Assessment

History

It is often difficult for the patient to localise pain, and the site may only be evident after careful examination. Patients tend to refer pain in the perineal region to the anus, but careful questioning often suggests it to be elsewhere, for example deep within the pelvis or over the coccyx. The word 'pain' has a variable meaning and it is important to distinguish discomfort from pain and to attempt to define the pain as mild or severe. The timing is also important, particularly the length of history, frequency of occurrence, periodicity and any relationship to defaecation.

Table 4.9. Perineal pain: Causes

Perianal	Thrombosed perianal varyx
	Fissure
	Condylomata acuminata
	Carcinoma
	Herpes simplex
	Chancre
Anal	Acute abscess ($\pm$ fistula)
	Chronic intersphincteric abscess
	Thrombosed prolapsed haemorrhoids
	Ulceration, e.g. in Crohn's disease
	Carcinoma
Rectal	Carcinoma
	Solitary ulcer
Pelvic floor	Proctalgia fugax
	Idiopathic pelvic pain
Non-anorectal	Gynaecological
	Urological
	Musculoskeletal
	Neurological

Severe pain is most commonly caused by an acute fissure, an anorectal abscess, a thrombosed perianal varyx or thrombosed prolapsed internal haemorrhoids. All are exacerbated by defaecation. The pain from a thrombosed varyx is constant and the patient can often be specific about the time of onset. Not uncommonly, it follows a bout of straining resulting in the sudden onset of a tender perineal lump, the pain of which persists for a few days before spontaneous resolution. An abscess causes a throbbing pain and in some cases there is a history of periodicity with attacks lasting a few days only to recur every few weeks or months; this suggests a chronic intersphincteric abscess or, if resolution of an exacerbation coincides with the discharge of pus, an established fistula-in-ano.

Pain from an anal fissure may also be periodic and usually occurs on defaecation, often persisting for some hours afterwards. Some minor bleeding is usual. Uncomplicated haemorrhoids rarely cause pain, which if present is more likely to be due to another lesion such as a fissure. Less common anal causes such as condylomata acuminata, herpes simplex, ulceration in Crohn's disease and carcinoma may be painful through ulceration, inflammation or secondary infection, or invasion of nerves.

Solitary ulcer sometimes causes a dull, persistent ache in the perineum and occasionally severe pain. Other symptoms include straining at stool and the passage of blood and mucus. Proctalgia fugax, which may be due to spasm of the pelvic floor muscles, is uncommon but recognisable by the typical nature of the pain. It occurs intermittently, perhaps every few weeks and often at night. The patient describes a cramp-like spasm deep within the perineum lasting for a few seconds to several minutes. It passes off spontaneously but can be extremely severe while it lasts.

A small group of unfortunate patients suffer from persistent pain in the anus or deep within the pelvis in the absence of any apparent lesion. Sometimes its original onset is stated to coincide with an episode of trauma—a pelvic operation, for example a hysterectomy, or treatment of an anal condition such as haemorrhoids or fissure. The pain may last for hours and be exacerbated by defaecation, it may have been present for years and can be completely disabling. Such patients often exhibit psychological abnormalities and many have symptoms typical of the irritable bowel syndrome. They may also complain of difficulty in evacuation and have abnormal perineal descent. The cause of the pain is unknown.

Examination

INSPECTION. A thrombosed varyx, anal fissure, perianal skin lesions and the external opening of a fistula are diagnosed on inspection. An acute abscess usually produces a perianal swelling with reddened oedematous overlying skin, but absence of such a swelling does not exclude the diagnosis since pus can track upwards without pointing in the perineum.

DIGITAL EXAMINATION AND SIGMOIDOSCOPY. If tolerated, an attempt is made to identify an area of tenderness or induration suggesting a localised lesion and to establish the presence or absence of proctitis. If too painful the examination can be deferred until the pain has settled, unless immediate action is necessary (for example with an abscess). Examination under anaesthetic is then indicated and any necessary treatment can also be carried out at the same time.

NON-ANORECTAL CAUSES. An enlarged uterus, tender cervix, abnormal prostate or a pelvic mass are indications of non-anorectal disease. There may be evidence of spinal disease and neurological abnormalities affecting the legs or perineum.

Investigation

Further tests include a plain X-ray film of the pelvis and spine, contrast radiculography and urological and gynaecological investigations as necessary in the individual case.

Patients with perineal pain in whom no obvious cause can be found can rarely be helped.

Diarrhoea

Most cases of diarrhoea are due to infective gastroenteritis or to functional bowel disease. However it is a common presentation of many forms of colorectal and some types of small bowel disease.

Differential Diagnosis

The causes of diarrhoea are given in Table 4.10. In inflammatory diseases diarrhoea is due to a combination of increased exudation of water from the mucosa, reduced reabsorption and irritability of the bowel leading to accelerated transit of increased volumes of liquid stool. Obstructing lesions sometimes also cause frequency but usually with the passage of small volumes of stool of fairly normal consistency. Some diseases can produce both diffuse inflammation and a localised stricture.

Antibiotics are a common cause of diarrhoea, either through hypersensitivity of the individual, or because they cause a change in the faecal flora: such a change occurs in pseudomembranous colitis, when suppression of normal intestinal bacteria favours growth of the pathogen *Clostridium difficile*. Laxative abuse is also common.

Alactasia is rare but important to identify, as a diet that excludes milk and milk products is effective treatment. The diarrhoea in this case is caused through the failure to split lactose, which consequently remains in the intestinal lumen and acts as an osmotic laxative. Bile salts are irritant to the colon and may cause diarrhoea after resection of the terminal ileum where they are normally reabsorbed. Diarrhoea may simply be due to the overproduction of mucus, for example by a neoplasm or solitary ulcer.

Table 4.10. Diarrhoea: Causes

Inflammation
Infective
Virus (rotavirus)
Bacteria (*Salmonella, Shigella, E. coli, Campylobacter, Clostridium difficile*)
Parasites (amoebiasis, giardiasis, strongyloidiasis)

Non-infective
Ulcerative colitis
Crohn's disease
Radiation enteritis
Ischaemic bowel disease

Motility disorder
Functional bowel disease
Diverticular disease

Mucus overproduction
Adenoma
Carcinoma
Solitary ulcer

Obstruction
Stricture: carcinoma, diverticular disease, Crohn's
    disease, radiation enteritis, ischaemic
bowel disease
Faecal impaction

Malabsorption
Coeliac disease
Internal fistula
Surgical resections
Pancreatic disease
Short bowel syndrome
Blind loop syndrome

Digestive failure
Alactasia

Metabolic disease
Thyrotoxicosis
Hormone-secreting tumours

Drugs
Laxatives
Antibiotics

Psychogenic causes
Anxiety

Clinical Assessment

History

The term diarrhoea may be used by patients to describe increased frequency of defaecation, loose consistency, urgency or incontinence, and each must be distinguished in the history. Frequent visits to the lavatory may not necessarily indicate diarrhoea. It may be, for example, that excessive mucus production or pus formation is the reason. In other cases such as the solitary ulcer syndrome there is often a frequent call to stool although actual defaecation does not occur with every attempt to pass stool. Urgency is defined as a sudden, rapidly increasing desire to defaecate which is often irresistible and may lead to incontinence. It is frequently the aspect of diarrhoea that patients find most hard to bear.

Diarrhoea may be episodic in conditions such as inflammatory bowel disease or functional bowel disease which tend to exacerbations and remissions.

PREDISPOSING FACTORS. Predisposing factors may include food poisoning, contact with other cases of diarrhoea or visits to areas where infective diarrhoea is endemic. There may be a history of previous intestinal operations or radiotherapy and a family history of inflammatory bowel disease or carcinoma may be relevant. Laxative-taking is sometimes denied by the patient.

OTHER SYMPTOMS. Blood and mucus in the faeces suggest some form of colorectal disease, which may also cause weight loss, anorexia and abdominal pain. Symptoms of thyrotoxicosis may be present. In partial obstruction (most commonly due to cancer) or faecal impaction, constipation and diarrhoea often occur together.

Examination and Investigation

LARGE BOWEL. A convenient order of examination and investigations is given in Table 4.11. Anorectal examination and barium enema examination with colonoscopy if indicated will identify most cases of non-infective large bowel disease. A stool sample must be obtained in every case at the initial consultation and it is wise to take a blood sample for serological tests if an infective cause is strongly suspected. Thyroid function tests should also be requested.

SMALL BOWEL. If these tests fail to make a diagnosis the small bowel should be investigated, at least by a small bowel meal. This will reveal any structural lesion and show abnormalities in some cases of coeliac disease. In suspected malabsorption faecal fat estimation, vitamin B12 absorption tests, estimation of serum and red cell folate levels and jejunal biopsy may be indicated. Alactasia is diagnosed by a lactose tolerance test.

OTHER INVESTIGATIONS. Examination of a duodenal aspirate is necessary for the diagnosis of *Strongyloides* infection. Phenolphthalein abuse can be detected by alkalinisation of the stool, which becomes pink. Gastrointestinal polypeptide hormone assays and investigations to locate a hormone-secreting tumour may be indicated.

Table 4.11. Diarrhoea: Diagnosis

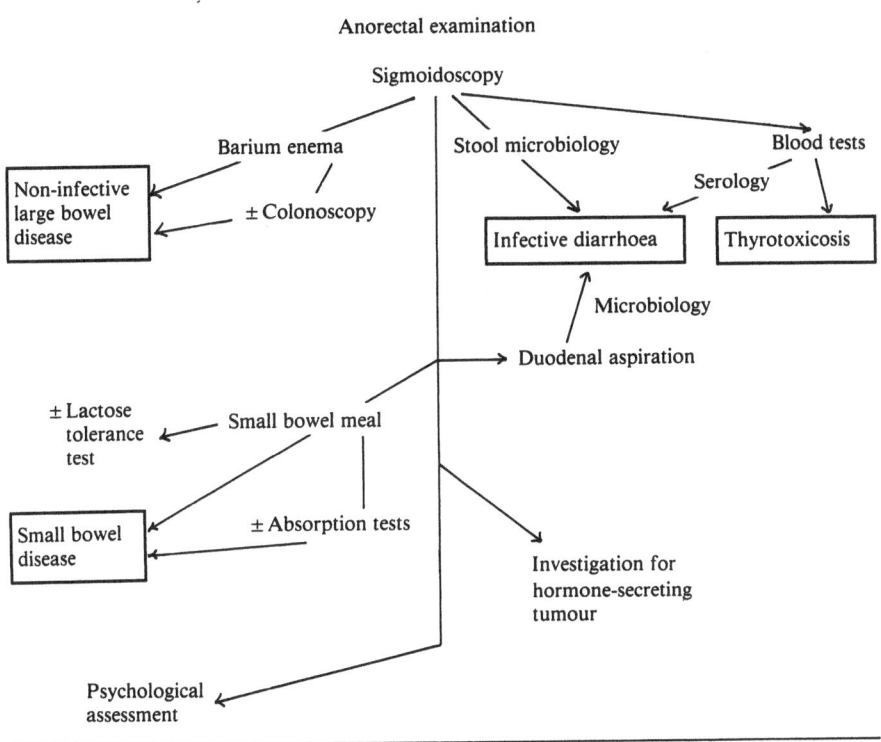

FUNCTIONAL DIARRHOEA. In many cases investigations are negative and a diagnosis of functional bowel disease is made by exclusion. Some of these patients show signs of anxiety but in the majority there seems to be no obvious psychological abnormality. The extent to which they should be investigated depends largely on the clinical assessment of the case after exclusion of the more common and serious causes of diarrhoea.

Constipation

Patients often consult their doctor complaining of 'constipation', using the term to mean an unsatisfactory bowel habit. Bowel habit can vary from the regular passage of a hard stool to the irregular or infrequent passage of a stool of normal consistency. Other symptoms such as abdominal distension, flatulence, headache and anorexia may be relieved by defaecation, leading the patient to believe he or she is constipated.

Differential Diagnosis (Table 4.12)

Constipation can be caused by a localised lesion producing a degree of obstruction or by some form of functional abnormality of the intestine leading to delayed transit. In some forms of functional constipation, for example aganglionosis or myxoedema, an underlying physical lesion can be found, but in the majority of cases there is no detectable morphological or hormonal abnormality. At the present time most forms of functional constipation can be classified only in terms of intestinal transit rates and the presence or absence of megacolon or megarectum.

In most people constipation is mild and is usually dietary or a manifestation of the irritable bowel syndrome. It is more severe in the minority with megacolon or in those with slow transit constipation. Patients with normal transit constipation appear to have a disorder of evacuation of the rectum and some may develop perineal descent and the solitary ulcer syndrome through excessive straining.

Table 4.12. Constipation: Causes

Localised lesion
Carcinoma
Diverticular disease
Crohn's disease
Other cause of stricture

Functional bowel disease
Megacolon: aganglionic
   Hirschsprung's disease
   Chagas' disease
Megacolon: idiopathic
   Megacolon
   Megarectum
Normal transit constipation
Slow transit constipation
Irritable bowel syndrome
Dietary constipation
Psychiatric (depression)
Pregnancy
Drugs
   Antidepressants
   Analgesics
   Iron
General medical diseases
   Myxoedema
   Diabetes mellitus
   Hypercalcaemia
   Uraemia
   Porphyria
Immobility

Clinical Assessment

History

Fewer than three evacuations per week is rare among apparently normal individuals. Patients with functional constipation often have a long history and a recent onset suggests an organic lesion, such as carcinoma. Constipation extending back to infancy raises the possibility of Hirschsprung's disease. Abdominal pain and distension often occur in patients with functional bowel disorders but the passage of blood suggests an organic cause.

Difficulty in evacuation with straining is often present in cases of idiopathic megacolon or megarectum. The condition usually starts in childhood or adolescence and is often associated with faecal impaction and with soiling (which does not occur in Hirschsprung's disease). There may be emotional and family problems and some patients are of low intelligence or have mental abnormalities.

In many patients with difficulty in defaecation there is no rectal or colonic distension but excessive straining at stool is common. Several visits to the lavatory may be made without a satisfactory evacuation. It is helpful to document the average number of visits per day and the time spent in the lavatory on each occasion.

A change in the patient's diet or lifestyle, for example a recent change to night-shift work, may be significant. Pregnancy and the possibility of general medical or psychiatric disease should be considered. Most antidepressants cause constipation. Radiological investigation is contraindicated in pregnancy unless it is essential in order to exclude a possibly serious illness.

Examination and Investigation (Table 4.13)

A localised lesion is excluded by anorectal examination and barium enema, and myxoedema, diabetes and pregnancy by blood and urine tests.

In patients with a functional disorder digital examination and sigmoidoscopy will determine whether the rectum is ballooned (as in megarectum) or collapsed (as in Hirschsprung's disease) and whether there is impaction. Melanosis coli is seen in patients who have taken laxatives for long periods: the mucosa has a dark-brown mottled appearance due to pigmentation, derived from metabolites of anthraquinones in macrophages in the submucosa.

The barium enema examination will distinguish between megacolon or megarectum and cases with a normal large bowel diameter. In patients with megacolon, tests of anorectal physiology are indicated. Absence of the rectosphincteric reflex is almost diagnostic of Hirschsprung's disease, the diagnosis being confirmed by a rectal biopsy taken just above the anorectal junction showing absent ganglia and increased numbers of cholinergic nerve fibres. If the reflex is present the diagnosis is idiopathic megacolon.

In patients shown to have a normal bowel calibre on barium enema examination, radiological transit studies will distinguish between normal and slow transit

Table 4.13. Constipation: Diagnosis

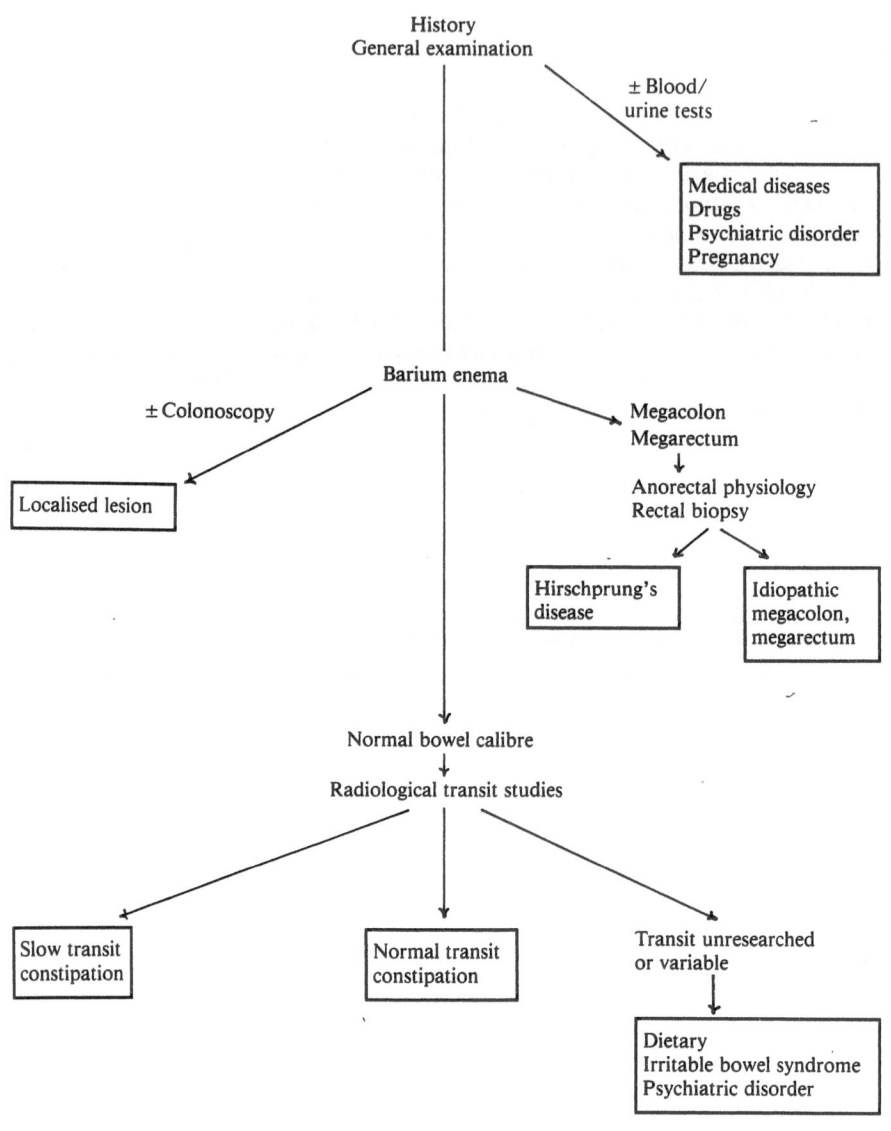

constipation. The patient takes a known number of radio-opaque pellets by mouth and a plain abdominal X-ray film is taken 5 days later. Slow transit is inferred if 20% or more of the markers are visible on the film. Tests to identify defaecation disorders include balloon evacuation studies with simultaneous measurement of intrarectal pressure during straining attempts to expel the balloon. At present they are mainly applicable to research.

Further Reading

Alexander S (1975) Dermatological aspects of anorectal disease. Clin Gastroenterol 4: 651–657

Allison DJ, Hemingway AP, Cunningham DA (1982) Angiography in gastrointestinal bleeding. Lancet II: 30–33

Baum S, Athanasoulis CA, Waltham AC (1974) Angiographic diagnosis and control of large-bowel bleeding. Dis Colon Rectum 17: 447–453

Behringer GE, Albright NL (1973) Diverticular disease of the colon. A frequent cause of massive rectal bleeding. Massachusetts General Hospital retrospective study. Am J Surg 125: 419–423

Colacchio TA, Forde KA, Patsos TJ, Nunez D (1982) Impact of modern diagnostic methods on the management of active rectal bleeding. Am J Surg 143: 607–610

Eyers AA, Thomson JPS (1979) Pruritus ani: is sphincter function important in aetiology? Lancet II: 1549–1551

Hunt R (1978) Rectal bleeding. Clin Gastroenterol 7: 719–740

Rahn NH, Tishler JM, Hau SY, Russinovitch NAE (1982) Diagnostic and interventional angiography in acute gastrointestinal hemorrhage. Radiology 143: 361–366

Read NW (ed) (1981) Diarrhoea: New insights. In: Clinical research reviews, vol 1, suppl 1.

Ryan P (1983) Changing concepts in diverticular disease. Dis Colon Rectum 26: 12–18

Sheedy PF, Fulton RE, Atwell DT (1975) Angiographic evaluation of patients with chronic gastrointestinal bleeding. Am J Roentgenol 123: 338–347

Silman AJ, Mitchell P, Nicholls RJ, Macrae FA, Leicester RJ, Bartram CI, Simmons MJ, Campbell PDJ, Hearn CED, Constable P (1983) Self-reported dark red bleeding as a marker comparable with occult blood testing in screening for large bowel neoplasms. Br J Surg 70: 721–724

Smith LE, Henrichs D, McCullah RD (1982) Prospective studies on etiology and treatment of pruritus ani. Dis Colon Rectum 25: 358–363

Swarbrick ET, Hunt RH, Fevre DI, Williams CB (1976) Colonoscopy for unexplained rectal bleeding. Gut 17: 823

Tedesco FJ, Waye JD, Raskin JB, Morris SJ, Greenwald RA (1978) Colonoscopic evaluation of rectal bleeding. A study of 304 patients. Ann Intern Med 89: 907–909

Waye JD, Braunfeld S (1982) Surveillance intervals after colonoscopic polypectomy. Endoscopy 14: 79–81

Williams CB, Macrae FA, Bartram CI (1982) A prospective study of diagnostic methods in adenoma follow-up. Endoscopy 14: 74–78

Williams CB, Thompson JPS (1977) Anorectal bleeding: A study of causes and investigative yields. Practitioner 219: 327–331

Winzelberg GG, Froelich JW, McKusick KA (1981) Radionuclide localisation of lower GI haemorrhage. Radiology 139: 465–469

5 Anal Disease

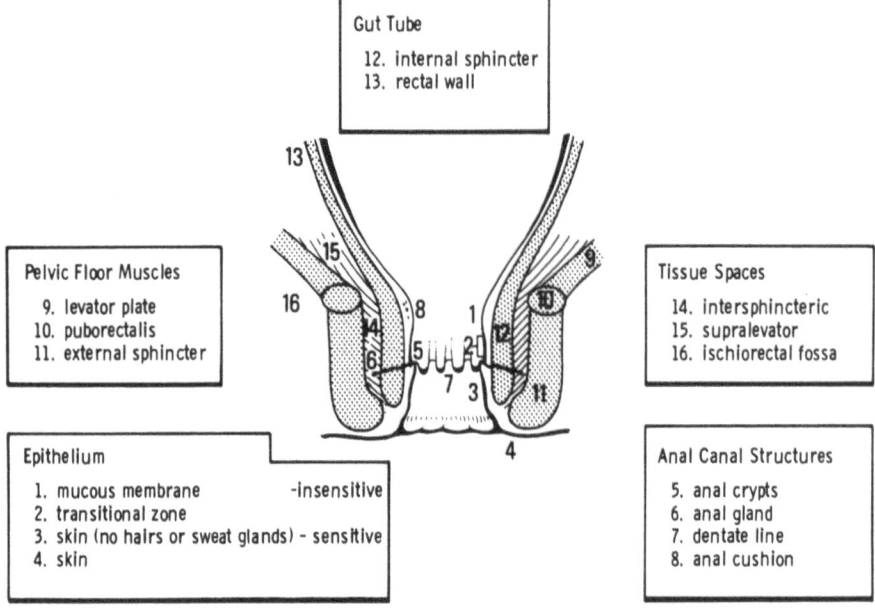

Fig. 5.1. Anal anatomy.

Gut Tube

12. internal sphincter
13. rectal wall

Pelvic Floor Muscles

9. levator plate
10. puborectalis
11. external sphincter

Tissue Spaces

14. intersphincteric
15. supralevator
16. ischiorectal fossa

Epithelium

1. mucous membrane   -insensitive
2. transitional zone
3. skin (no hairs or sweat glands) – sensitive
4. skin

Anal Canal Structures

5. anal crypts
6. anal gland
7. dentate line
8. anal cushion

Fissure-in-ano

Anal fissure occurs predominantly in young adults but it is sometimes seen in infants and children. It is a longitudinal ulcer in the skin-lined part of the anal

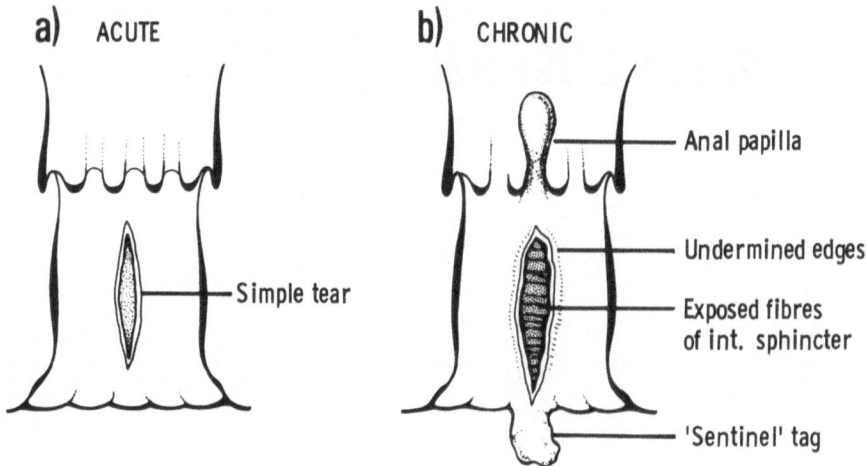

Fig. 5.2a, b. Clinical types of anal fissure.

canal which probably starts as a simple tear. The edges become undermined and the base deepens to expose the circular fibres of the internal sphincter (Fig. 5.2). An anal papilla may develop at the level of the dentate line and a redundant skin tag at the distal end of the fissure (sentinel pile). Fissure is associated with a low fistula-in-ano or intersphincteric abscess in 5%–10% of cases and is the commonest anal lesion associated with Crohn's disease.

The aetiology is unknown. It is often suggested that fissure is caused by the passage of a hard stool, but patients often do not have constipation and fissure may occur with diarrhoea. Resting anal pressure is raised in most cases but this may be due to secondary sphincter spasm induced by pain rather than to a primary sphincter disorder. Fissure may be the result of crypt infection as suggested by its association with anorectal sepsis and the similar midline distribution of fissure and internal openings. It often occurs in pregnancy.

Diagnosis

Symptoms

The incidence of symptoms is shown in Table 5.1. Almost all patients have pain and bleeding. Pain occurs during defaecation and often lasts for an hour or so afterwards; it can range from mild to very severe. Blood is usually seen as a smear on the toilet paper and is bright. Pruritus is common but constipation is present in only about one-quarter of cases. There may be a history of relapses and remissions indicating intermittent healing.

Table 5.1. Fissure-in-ano: Incidence of symptoms (%)

Pain	90
Bleeding	85
Pruritus	50
Constipation	25
Discharge	20

Signs

A fissure is diagnosed by inspection, parting the anal verge to show a longitudinal split in the lower anal canal. It occurs in the posterior midline in about 80% of cases and in almost all the remainder it is anterior; lateral fissures are rare. Occasionally both an anterior and posterior fissure are present. An anterior fissure is more common in females than in males.

In 20% of cases a simple split is the only physical sign, but in others a sentinel tag, anal papilla or a deep undermined ulcer may be present and are evidence of chronicity. It is usually possible to pass the paediatric sigmoidoscope without undue pain, enabling examination of the lower rectum to exclude proctitis.

Differential Diagnosis

A thrombosed perianal varyx or anorectal abscess may present with severe pain and a chronic intersphincteric abscess or intermittently discharging fistula may produce exacerbations and remissions similar to a long-standing fissure. Other causes of pain or discomfort include sexually transmitted diseases (such as warts, syphilitic lesions or herpes) and anal carcinoma. Bleeding may be due to haemorrhoids, proctitis or a low-lying rectal neoplasm.

The appearance of a syphilitic ulcer may be indistinguishable from an anal fissure but relative painlessness, atypical site and the presence of exudate causing matting of hairs should arouse suspicion.

Conditions associated with fissure, including anorectal sepsis, inflammatory bowel disease (especially Crohn's disease), anorectal tuberculosis, syphilis and Paget's disease of the anus, should be excluded by full anorectal examination and further investigation.

Investigation

Serological tests should be requested if syphilis is suspected. In patients with proctitis a rectal biopsy, microbiological examination of the stool and contrast radiology are indicated.

Table 5.2. Fissure-in-ano: Management

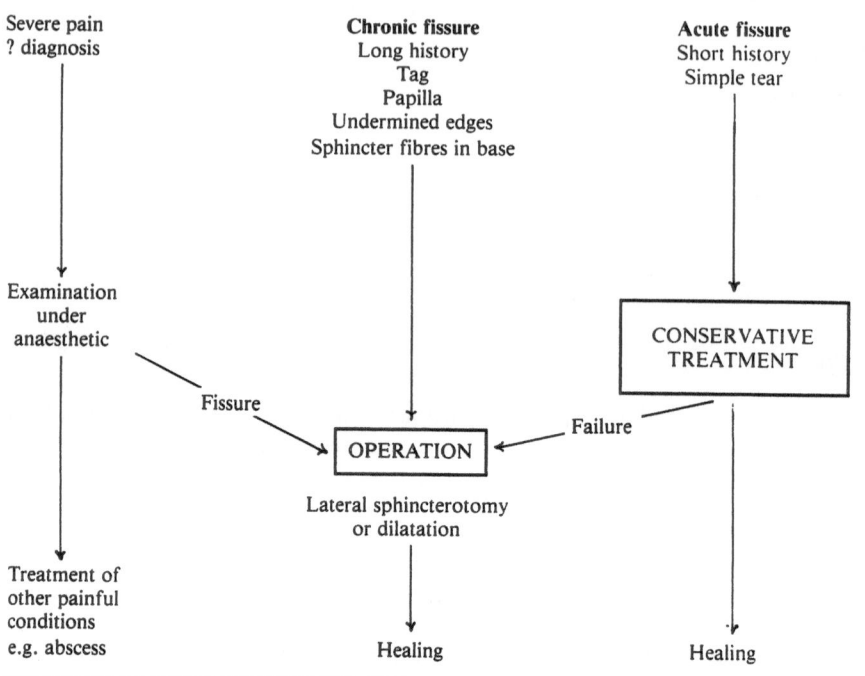

Management (Table 5.2)

Operative Treatment

INDICATIONS. Opinions on management may differ, but few would argue that a patient with severe pain should be operated on directly. This is better carried out with the patient under general rather than local anaesthesia since a more thorough examination of the anorectal region is afforded. Sigmoidoscopy can be performed without pain and associated conditions such as fistula excluded. It may be that the diagnosis is an anorectal abscess rather than a fissure, in which case the treatment is drainage.

Operation is also indicated in patients with a history of more than a few weeks or signs of chronicity. Conservative treatment in this group is usually ineffective. CHOICE OF OPERATION. The choice of operation lies between internal sphincterotomy and anal dilatation. Other treatments such as excision of the fissure or injection with sclerosant are used by some surgeons, but the good results obtained particularly by sphincterotomy strongly favour its adoption. *Lateral Sphincterotomy* (Fig. 5.3). Results are better when the operation is carried out with the patient under general rather than local anaesthesia. The

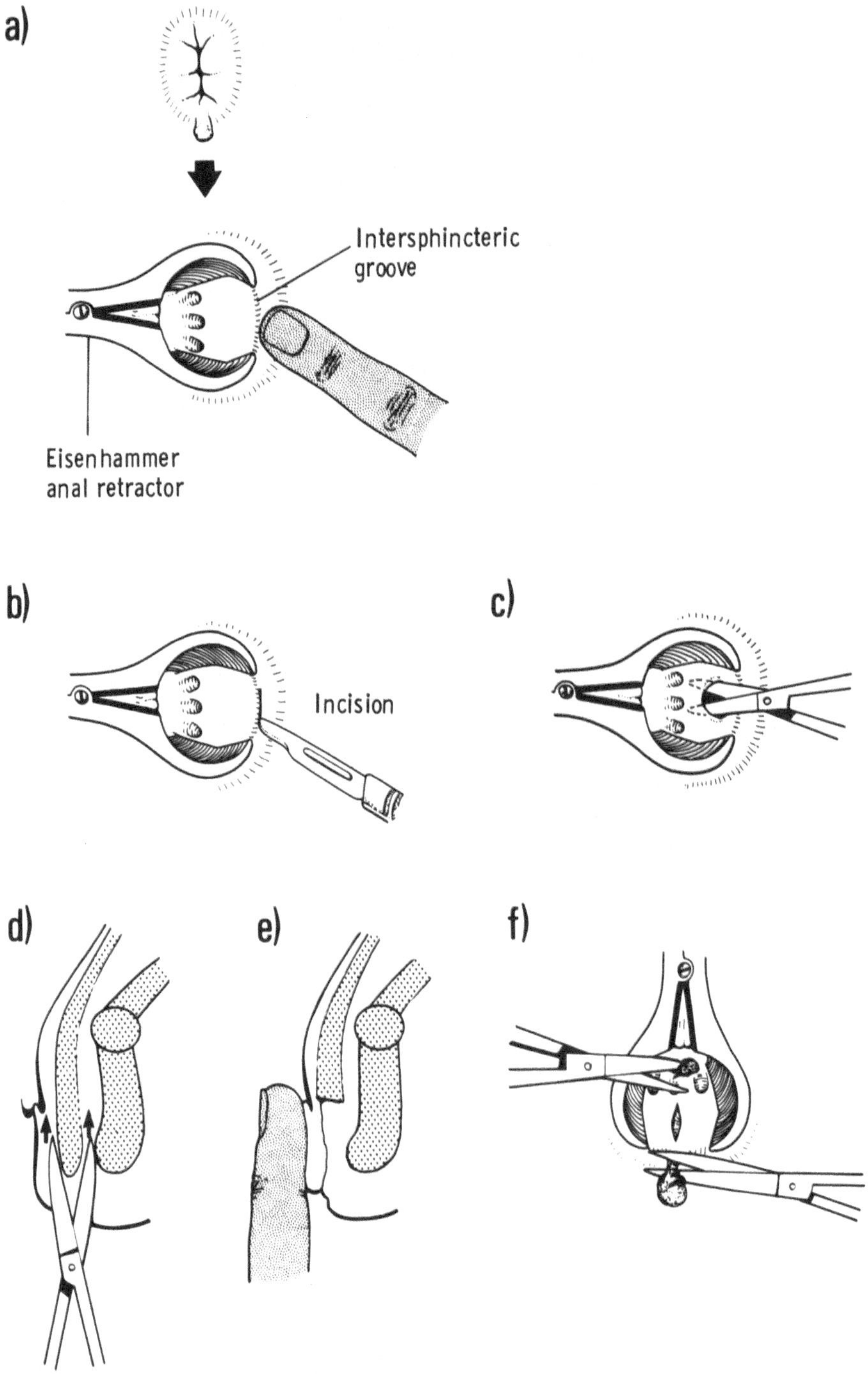

a)

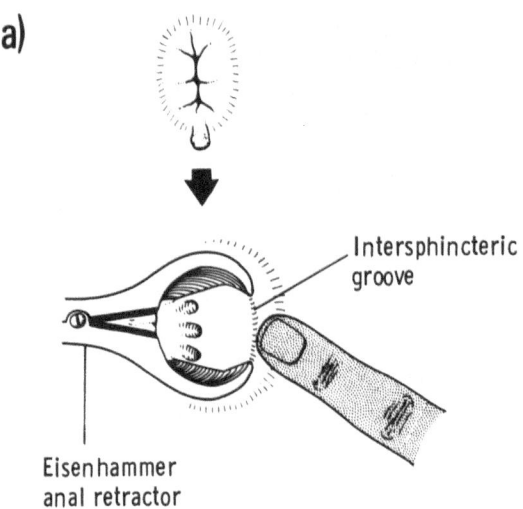

Intersphincteric
groove

Eisenhammer
anal retractor

b)   c)

Incision

d)   e)   f)

Fig. 5.3a–f. Lateral anal sphincterotomy for anal fissure.

operation includes division of the internal sphincter to the dentate line and excision of the sentinel tag and anal papilla. The fissure itself is not excised.

An anal retractor is inserted and opened, tensing the internal sphincter to demonstrate its lower border and the intersphincteric groove. A short circumferential incision is made laterally in the intersphincteric groove and the lower border of the internal sphincter is identified either by palpation or on direct vision, the fibres being white when compared with the brown-red colour of the external sphincter. The sphincter is mobilised by scissor dissection in the submucosal and intersphincteric planes and then divided up to the dentate line. Local pressure is applied for a minute or so for haemostasis and the skin wound is sutured with fine catgut or left open.

After lateral sphincterotomy, a V-shaped defect in the internal sphincter can be felt. Occasionally the mucosa is perforated and should be repaired by fine catgut. The tag and papilla are then removed and a gentle pressure dressing is applied and a bulk laxative prescribed.

Complications include bleeding, haematoma and rarely abscess and fistula formation. Minor disturbances of continence have been reported in about 5% of cases. Pain relief is often immediate and the fissure heals within 2–4 weeks.

Posterior Sphincterotomy. Posterior sphincterotomy used to be commonly practised but is now less popular as the functional results are poor compared with lateral sphincterotomy. Minor disturbances of continence have been reported in 20%–40% of cases. It is thought that these may be due to the posterior groove-like or 'key-hole' deformity produced by the operation acting as a channel down which mucus and occasionally small amounts of liquid faeces can seep. A posterior sphincterotomy will, however, be necessary where a fissure is associated with a posterior fistula or intersphincteric abscess.

Anal Stretch. In this operation the anus is dilated to admit four fingers. General anaesthesia is required and the dilatation is started by inserting one index finger followed gently by the other. A minute or so later both middle fingers are added and the dilatation is continued for about 5 minutes. A bulk laxative is prescribed postoperatively.

RESULTS. A summary of the results of various procedures is given in Tables 5.3, but this includes only one randomised trial. Lateral sphincterotomy appears to be superior in terms of both recurrence and continence, but it must be conceded that the only prospective clinical trial comparing lateral sphincterotomy with anal dilatation has reported lower recurrence rates for the latter. The high recurrence after lateral sphincterotomy (16%) in this study may have been because the operation was performed under local rather than general anaesthesia.

Conservative Treatment

Many surgeons treat all fissures by operation, but there is a group of patients in whom conservative treatment still has a place. These include those with a short history and in whom the fissure appears to be a simple, superficial split without a tag or papilla.

Table 5.3. Fissure-in-ano: Results of surgical treatment

	No. of patients	Persistence/ recurrence (%)	Disturbance of continence (%)
Lateral sphincterotomy			
Notaras (1971)[a]	82	0	6
Millar (1971)	105	0	3
Hoffman & Goligher (1970)	99	2	12
Hawley (1969)	24	0	0
Marby et al. (1979)[b]	75	16	–
Posterior sphincterotomy			
Bennett & Goligher (1962)	127	7	43
Magee et al. (1966)	139	3	20–30
Hawley (1969)	32	8	6
Anal dilatation			
Graham Stuart et al. (1961)	37	10	–
Watts et al. (1964)	95	16	28
Hawley (1969)	18	28	0
Marby et al. (1979)[b]	77	5	–

[a] For full details of references see pp.123–124.
[b] Randomised controlled trial.

The regimen consists of a bulk laxative to soften the stool and a local anaesthetic preparation to relieve pain. There is no evidence that an anal dilator reduces the failure rate of conservative treatment and there is therefore no justification for its use.

Healing within a few weeks occurs in about 50% of cases and appears to be maintained in almost all when followed for at least one year. There is no evidence that the regimen per se is responsible and it is quite likely that healing is spontaneous. If improvement has not occurred after 2–3 weeks then conservative treatment should be abandoned and the patient referred for operation. Local anaesthetics can cause contact dermatitis and should not be used for long periods.

Haemorrhoids

Haemorrhoids account for symptoms in over half the patients presenting to a rectal clinic, but they can also be demonstrated in many with other diseases. The diagnosis and management should therefore be guided by two principles: first colonic or rectal disease must be excluded and secondly asymptomatic haemorrhoids should not be treated. Under no circumstances should treatment be given without discussing the options with the patient beforehand.

Definition

A haemorrhoid consists of an internal and external component. The internal component is located in the anal canal above the dentate line and is formed by blood vessels, connective tissue and smooth muscle covered by mucosa. The external component is located at the anal verge and consists of blood vessels forming the perianal subcutaneous venous plexus covered by skin. The two components are in vascular communication.

It has been postulated that internal haemorrhoids are due to enlargement of the anal cushions, which are normal structures, lying in the upper anal canal, composed of the same tissues and believed to contribute to anal canal closure by their apposition with each other. Two factors have been proposed to explain their enlargement, namely distal sliding of the anal canal lining and venous congestion. Both may occur from straining at stool (often admitted to by the patient) and venous congestion may in addition be due to the constricting action of the anal sphincter or to impedance of venous return, for example by pelvic tumours (including a gravid uterus). Resting anal canal pressure is raised in patients with haemorrhoids and there is histological evidence of hypertrophy of the external sphincter muscle fibres. Sliding leads to stretching and attenuation of the connective tissue within the anal cushion, causing it to become redundant; it also accounts for enlargement of the external component through subluxation of the cutaneous lining of the lower anal canal.

Diagnosis

Symptoms

Haemorrhoids may cause almost any anal symptoms but the commonest are bleeding, prolapse discomfort and pruritus ani (Table 5.4). Bleeding is usually bright and separate from the stool, often dripping immediately after defaecation. Occasionally, however, it is dark if the blood has been retained in the rectum for any length of time.

Prolapse probably indicates a more advanced stage of the disease. Its severity can be gauged by establishing the timing and duration. Prolapse may occur only during defaecation and retract spontaneously afterwards, it may require replacement by the patient or it may be present all the time. Prolapse may be confused with perianal swelling caused by the external haemorrhoidal component.

Table 5.4. Haemorrhoids: Incidence of symptoms (50 consecutive patients)

	Prevalence (%)	Most troublesome symptom (%)
Bleeding	81	33
Discomfort	64	17
Pruritus	62	6
Prolapse	50	22
Swelling	47	2
Pain	35	19
Discharge	29	1

Discomfort is common particularly when there is prolapse. It may be described as a feeling of fullness in the perineum or anus or as a sensation similar to the desire to defaecate. Often the patient strains excessively in an attempt to get relief, making the haemorrhoids worse. Pain may occur even in the absence of acute thrombosis or strangulation, but it may alternatively indicate the presence of a coexisting painful anal lesion such as fissure, abscess or a thrombosed perianal varyx.

Haemorrhoids, especially if prolapsing, often cause a mucous discharge which in turn may lead to pruritus by producing maceration of the perianal skin. Anal hygiene is difficult when there is a large external component and the patient may therefore suffer from faecal soiling.

Symptoms of haemorrhoids come and go with spontaneous exacerbations and remissions. Bleeding in particular may occur in episodes which resolve completely for weeks, months or even years. The frequency of symptoms is a factor in deciding treatment and this cyclical behaviour should also be borne in mind when assessing the results.

Signs

Haemorrhoids are diagnosed by inspection, which should be carried out first with the patient at rest and then during straining. On inspection of the perineum the enlarged external component and any prolapsed internal haemorrhoids will be seen. Proctoscopy will reveal swelling (the normal anal cushions) in the right anterior, right posterior and left lateral position in any normal individual, and it may be difficult in an individual case to decide whether they are sufficiently large to be diagnosed as haemorrhoids. However, enlargement can be inferred if they bulge into the lumen of the proctoscope. The mucosa over a haemorrhoid is often reddened and may be bleeding. Sometimes areas of white plaque formation are seen on its surface. This is due to squamous metaplasia of the mucosa caused by trauma and is diagnostic of repeated prolapse.

Differential Diagnosis

In most patients straining during proctoscopy causes the mucosa of the lower rectum to descend to just above the anorectal ring. This is most clearly seen anteriorly and some degree of descent appears to be a normal finding. It can be so marked, however, as to enter the proctoscope or even to appear at the anal verge on direct inspection of the perineum. The term anterior mucosal prolapse is applied to this condition, which causes symptoms identical to haemorrhoids and is often associated. A complete rectal prolapse may also produce similar symptoms. The differential diagnosis also includes any condition causing bleeding or a lump or pain at the anus. A carcinoma is the most important condition to keep in mind.

An adequate sigmoidoscopy must be carried out in all patients and full investigation of the large bowel is indicated if there is uncertainty whether

symptoms are due to haemorrhoids. Flexible sigmoidoscopy is particularly useful
in this situation. Anal manometry has been recommended by some for selecting
patients for treatment, but it is doubtful whether this investigation is useful.

Management

In recent years there has been a marked trend away from haemorrhoidectomy to
more conservative methods of treatment and at present only about 5%-10% of
patients in Britain are treated by this operation. Change has largely been due to
the development of a variety of relatively simple techniques suitable for outpatient or day case management. Injection treatment has been in use since the last
century but rubber band ligation, maximal anal dilation, cryotherapy, infrared
coagulation and lateral sphincterotomy are products of the last 30 years.

The choice of treatment depends on the type of symptom, its frequency and
severity and the preference of the doctor.

Classification

The traditional staging of haemorrhoids does not distinguish patients with
occasional and mild symptoms from those with persistent trouble. It also fails to
identify the relatively small group of patients in whom haemorrhoidectomy is the
only feasible method of treatment. A classification with four subgroups gives a
more useful guide to treatment (Table 5.5).

Table 5.5. Haemorrhoids: Clinical classification and choice of treatment

Classification	Symptoms	Treatment[a]
Group 1	Occasional symptoms	Reassurance after exclusion of colorectal disease
Group 2	Bleeding; no prolapse	**Injection** Rubber band ligation (Infrared coagulation) (Cryotherapy)
Group 3	Prolapse	**Rubber band ligation** Injection (Infrared coagulation) (Cryotherapy)
Group 4	Prolapse and large symptomatic external component	Haemorrhoidectomy

[a] Avoidance of straining; bulk laxatives in all cases.

GROUP 1 (occasional mild symptoms). About 10%-15% of the normal adult
population will have had an episode of anal bleeding within the previous year.
Some may present to their general practitioner and by the time they are seen in
hospital the episode is long past. Their motive for seeking medical advice is

usually the fear of cancer. Reassurance can only be given if the doctor is confident that the colon and rectum are normal, and further investigation, especially in older patients, may be necessary. Often the diagnosis of haemorrhoids can only be presumed after negative investigation. In these patients local treatment of haemorrhoids is probably unnecessary and advice to avoid straining or constipation (e.g. by taking bran or a bulk laxative if necessary) is all that is required. The patient must not, however, be made to feel that he or she has wasted the doctor's time and should be commended for coming forward for examination and advised to return if worried or if symptoms recur.

GROUP 2 (troublesome bleeding). This group includes patients in whom bleeding is recurrent, perhaps every few weeks or months, but prolapse is absent. Treatment is necesssary and may include bulk laxatives, injection, rubber band ligation, infrared coagulation or cryosurgery.

GROUP 3 (prolapse). Provided prolapse is due to the internal component any of the outpatient methods can be applied and haemorrhoidectomy reserved for those in whom conservative treatment, perhaps after trying several different techniques, has failed. Rubber band ligation is more logical than injection since tissue is actually removed.

GROUP 4 (prolapse with large symptomatic external component). Patients who have prolapsing internal haemorrhoids and an external component causing symptoms are unsuitable for rubber band ligation or injection treatment owing to the rich sensory nerve supply of the skin. Haemorrhoidectomy offers the only prospect of cure.

Methods

LOCAL PREPARATIONS. Many patients treat themselves with preparations purchased from commercial pharmacists. These include creams, ointments, jellies and suppositories often containing a steroid preparation combined with a local anaesthetic or hydroxyethylrutosides (vasoactive drugs with an anti-inflammatory action said to increase capillary permeability). There is no evidence that any of these agents is effective, and it is likely that any improvement is simply due to spontaneous remission. Self treatment may delay the diagnosis of serious disease such as cancer and can therefore be dangerous.

INJECTION SCLEROTHERAPY (Fig. 5.4). A sclerosing liquid is injected into the submucosa around the vascular pedicle of the haemorrhoid at the level of the anorectal ring. Inflammation with subsequent fibrosis around the blood vessels leads, it is believed, to a reduction of blood supply to the haemorrhoid and also fixation of the mucosa reducing the tendency to prolapse. Various substances are used, including phenol (5%) in arachis oil, quinine (20%) or sodium tetradecate. With the last the aim is to provoke thrombosis within the haemorrhoid.

A proctoscope is passed into the rectum and withdrawn slowly until the haemorrhoids begin to bulge into the lumen. The instrument is then tilted towards the haemorrhoid to be injected and advanced a few millimetres just above its base, i.e. at the level of the anorectal junction. The needle is introduced into the submucosa at this point and about 3–6 ml of sclerosant are slowly

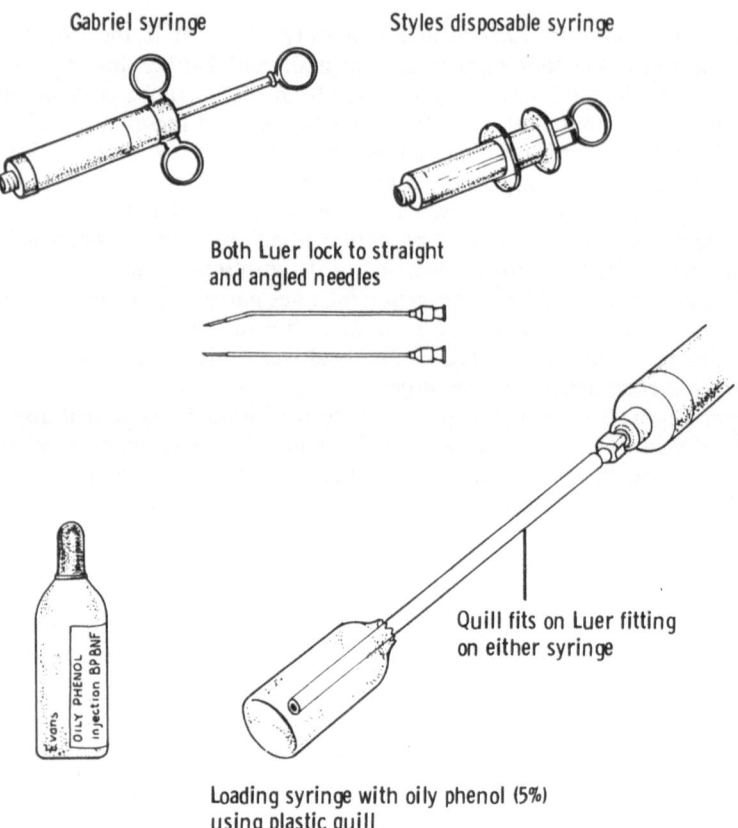

Gabriel syringe   Styles disposable syringe

Both Luer lock to straight
and angled needles

Quill fits on Luer fitting
on either syringe

Loading syringe with oily phenol (5%)
using plastic quill

Fig. 5.4. Equipment required for injection sclerotherapy.

injected (Fig. 5.5). No resistance should be felt unless a previous injection has been given. The sign of a correctly placed injection is the appearance of submucosal vessels on the bleb of mucosa raised by the injection. The needle is left in place for at least 10 seconds after injecting and is then withdrawn. Each haemorrhoid is treated in turn, but it is wise to inject the right posterior haemorrhoid first, since it is the most difficult.

In male patients care must be taken when injecting into the anterior haemorrhoid since accidental injection into the prostate gland is a danger. An Abel proctoscope designed with a slot in the side to allow the haemorrhoid to bulge into the lumen of the instrument may be of value, especially in treating patients who have had previous injections.

It requires practice to become competent at this technique and some of the problems encountered and suggestions for solving them are given in Table 5.6.

The patient should be warned that a small amount of bleeding may occur during the subsequent few hours and is also advised to take a laxative for 24–48 hours. Usually time off work is not necessary. Some discomfort is felt during the

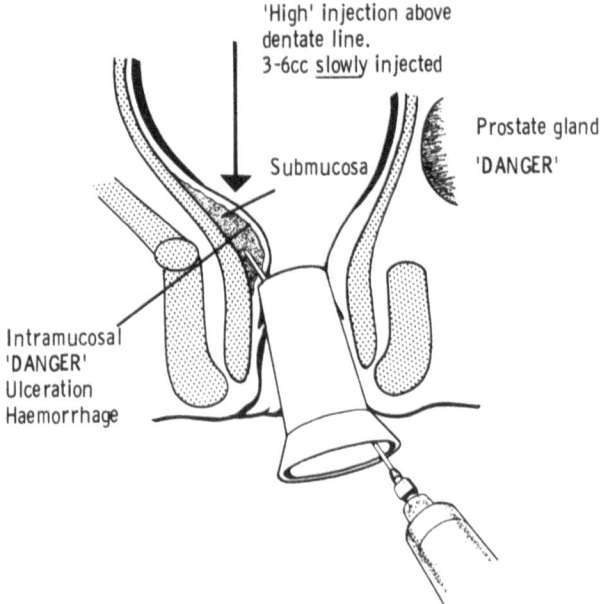

'High' injection above
dentate line.
3-6cc slowly injected

Prostate gland
'DANGER'

Submucosa

Intramucosal
'DANGER'
Ulceration
Haemorrhage

Fig. 5.5. Technique of injection sclerotherapy.

subsequent few days in about 20%–50% of patients but pain is less common (5%–20%). Secondary haemorrhage is rare and is usually associated with ulceration at the injection site. A second visit at 2 months is arranged, at which the injection is repeated only if symptoms are still present.

Table 5.6. Haemorrhoids: Technical difficulties of injection

Problem	Cause	Remedy
Difficult exposure	Proctoscope at wrong angle	Angulate proctoscope or withdraw and re-insert
	Faeces, blood	Swab
Difficulty in piercing mucosa	Blunt needle	Change
	Site of previous injection	Try different site
Resistance on injection	Previous injection	Try different site
	Blocked needle	Check
	Injection too deep	Withdraw
Mucosa goes white	Injection too superficial	Advance
Pain	Injection too deep	Stop
	Injection too distal	Stop
Solution leaks out after withdrawing needle	Injection too rapid	Inject slower. Leave needle in place for 10 seconds
Bleeding after injection	Traumatised submucosal vessel	Apply topical adrenaline solution (1:1000)

RUBBER BAND LIGATION (Fig. 5.6). The aim is to place a rubber band at the base of the haemorrhoid which first reduces blood flow by snaring the feeding vessel, secondly removes some of the haemorrhoid's bulk, and thirdly causes fibrosis at the point of banding to fix the mucosa and impede prolapse.

The instrument consists of two concentric cylinders which move over each other. The cylinders are mounted on independent shafts, one running within the other. The handle is constructed to allow the operator to move the outer cylinder forward on the inner using one hand. A rubber band mounted on the inner cylinder can thus be eased off its end. The loaded instrument is introduced through the proctoscope which is held steady by a nurse or the patient and the mucosa at the upper level of the haemorrhoid is grasped gently with crocodile forceps passed up through the inner cylinder. A tongue of mucosa is brought into

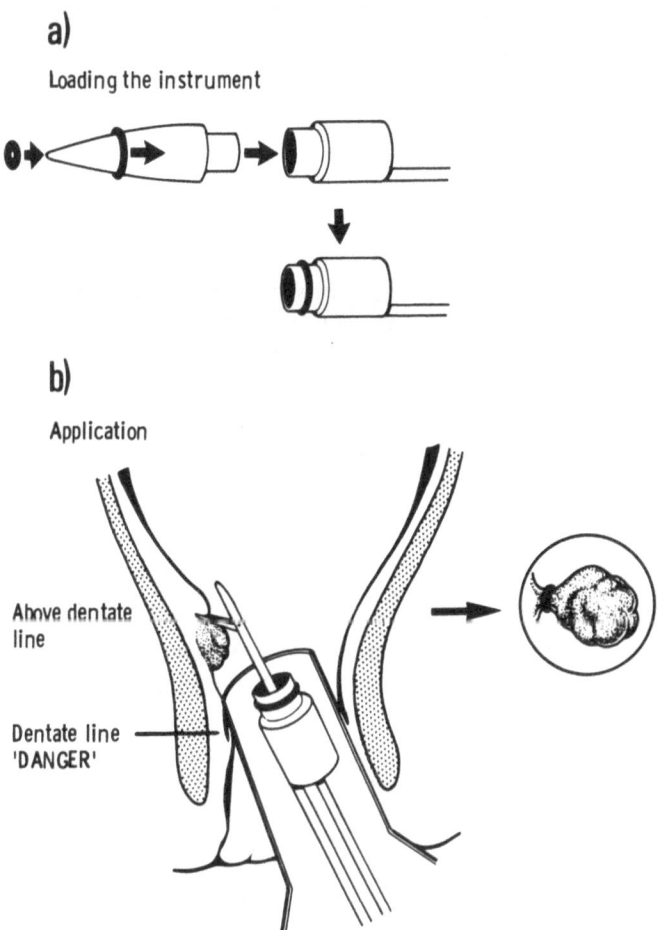

Fig. 5.6a, b. Technique of rubber band ligation.

the inner cylinder by traction. The patient must be asked at this stage whether pain is felt. If not, the rubber band is released when as much mucosa as feasible has been drawn down. Under no circumstances should the band be applied if grasping the mucosa is painful, and it should never be placed near the dentate line.

The strangulated tissue becomes necrotic and sloughs within a few days and the wound heals by fibrosis. At least two haemorrhoids can be treated at one session. The patient should be given a mild laxative for a few days.

The cardinal rule of banding haemorrhoids is to ensure that tissue which has tactile sensation is not incorporated. A band which causes immediate pain should be removed straightaway. This can be done through a proctoscope using a fine scalpel, but removal is only rarely necessary

The two commonest complications are pain and bleeding. Some degree of discomfort is experienced by a quarter to half of patients and they should be warned that this may occur. In about 10% pain is severe and may render the patient unable to work. Sometimes this comes on after an interval of a few days and is often due to the development of a thrombosed external varyx. Secondary haemorrhage occurs in about 2%–5% of cases. This can be severe and may require admission to hospital. The patient should be sensibly warned of the possibility of some bleeding and advised to seek medical advice if this occurs.

INFRARED COAGULATION (Fig. 5.7). A controlled area of heat coagulation is produced in the vascular pedicle of the haemorrhoid using an infrared source. The principle is similar to injection sclerotherapy and the site of the application identical. Tissue destruction occurs to a depth of 3 mm and is thought to cause direct damage to the feeding blood vessels and fixation of the mucosa as the defect heals by scarring.

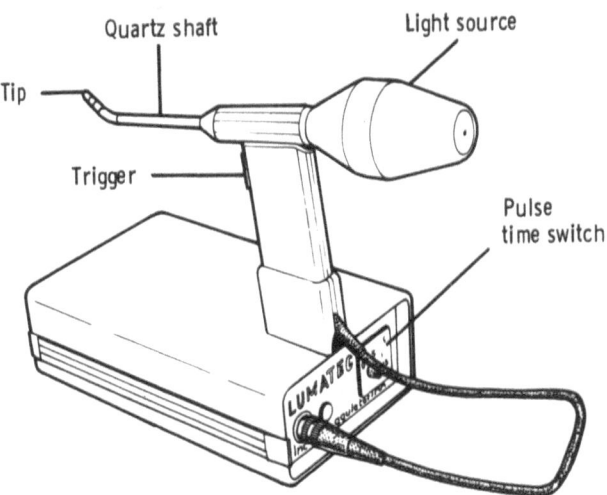

Fig. 5.7. The infrared coagulator.

The apparatus consists of a power source connected to a pistol. A tungsten-halogen bulb (14 watt) in the head of the pistol is activated by a trigger switch and the infrared irradiation produced is concentrated along a quartz fibre shaft to its tip. A switch on the power source allows the duration of exposure to be adjusted between 0.5 and 2.0 seconds.

A proctoscope is passed and the mucosa just above the haemorrhoid to be treated is identified. The pistol is held in the right hand and the shaft advanced so that its tip makes direct contact with the selected area. With the instrument set to a 1 second exposure, the trigger is pressed. Two applications per haemorrhoid have been used with no apparent adverse effect. No special after-care is required.

Pain occurs in about 5% of cases and minor bleeding in about 10%–22%, but secondary haemorrhage is uncommon.

CRYOHAEMORRHOIDECTOMY. The haemorrhoid is treated by freezing to cause necrosis and sloughing, with healing of the resulting wound by secondary intention. In contrast to other outpatient methods cryotherapy has been used to treat the external as well as the internal component and in these circumstances should be regarded as equivalent to surgical haemorrhoidectomy. The treatment may, however, be applied selectively to the internal haemorrhoids, and can then be more aptly compared with injection, rubber band ligation or infrared coagulation.

Freezing is achieved by contact with a probe cooled either by liquid nitrous oxide (boiling point − 70 °C) or nitrogen (boiling point − 180 °C). The probe is connected to a cylinder containing the liquid and flow to the tip is switched on and off by a trigger on the probe.

Some surgeons use local anaesthesia for cryohaemorrhoidectomy. A proctoscope is passed and the tip of the probe is applied to the haemorrhoid. The trigger is pressed until the tissue is seen to freeze into a so-called ice ball; this usually takes 30–90 seconds. The trigger is released and the probe removed as the tissue thaws. After 1–2 days the swelling resembles a strangulated thrombosed haemorrhoid and by about a week sloughing has occurred. Discharge is common especially if the wound is external and healing may take several weeks.

Cryotherapy was more popular 10 years ago than today. The disadvantages of the method are due to the uncontrolled extent of destruction (which fairly often leaves residual skin tags and haemorrhoids) and to the morbidity of the wound. The initial reports of cryohaemorrhoidectomy made little mention of pain, discharge and delayed healing, but more recent published series show that they are common. It seems, however, that fewer unwanted effects occur when, as with injection or rubber band ligation, treatment is confined to the internal haemorrhoids.

MANUAL DILATATION. The rationale is to reduce resting anal canal pressure, which may be raised in haemorrhoids and is considered by some to be a causative factor.

The operation is carried out under general anaesthesia but the patient is able to go home the same day. Dilation is performed slowly over 5–10 minutes until the anus admits 8 fingers. Pressure should be applied laterally away from the weaker anterior and posterior poles of the anus. A large pack is left in the anal canal and removed an hour later. Postoperatively the patient is given a bulk laxative and is instructed to pass a special dilator for 1 minute at a time according to the following regime: every evening for 2 weeks, alternate evenings for 2 weeks, once a week for up to 2 months and once a month for up to 6 months.

Complications include local bruising and occasionally faecal incontinence. It is difficult from published accounts to know how often difficulty in holding flatus occurs, but it would be surprising if it were not at least as common as after anal stretching for fissure (20%–30%). Anal dilatation is unwise in the elderly, particularly women in whom the anal sphincter may already be weak, since incontinence is more likely and is difficult to treat.

SPHINCTEROTOMY. Sphincterotomy, both lateral and posterior, has been used to reduce anal pressure but the results are poor.

HAEMORRHOIDECTOMY. Various techniques are described in surgical textbooks.

Results

The results are now available of many trials that compare outpatient treatments for haemorrhoids, but almost all lack comparison with a non-treated control group. Such a control is important owing to the periodic nature of haemorrhoidal symptoms—particularly bleeding, which has been reported to stop spontaneously in up to 60% of patients followed over several months without treatment. This high resolution rate is comparable to many of the results reported after active treatment. In assessing results it is also important to follow the patient for a sufficient period of time. In general, symptomatic improvement noted after a few months falls by 15%–30% when the patients are seen at 1 year. Bleeding haemorrhoids often cause other symptoms and it is inevitable that in many trials haemorrhoids of different stages are included in the same treatment group. Assessment of results is also difficult owing to the subjective nature of the disease; and in some trials bleeding and prolapse are not distinguished.

The results of a selection of recent trials are given in Table 5.7. They are all prospective and with one exception patients have been randomised to the treatment received. The following conclusions are drawn:

The results for a given treatment vary considerably.

There is little difference between injection, rubber band ligation and infrared coagulation for bleeding, but rubber band ligation is superior to injection and probably to infrared coagulation for prolapse (Table 5.8).

The results of manual dilation, although excellent in the one uncontrolled study, are no better than rubber band ligation for bleeding and appear to be worse for prolapse.

Sphincterotomy gives poor results.

Cryotherapy gives poorer results than rubber band ligation in the only trial where these are compared. However it is as good as haemorrhoidectomy in another trial.

Haemorrhoidectomy gives better results than injection, rubber band ligation and manual dilation.

Table 5.7. Haemorrhoids: Results of clinical trials

	Follow-up (months)	Symptom	No. of asymptomatic patients/no. of patients followed[a]						
			Injection	RBL	MDA	IR	C	LS	H
Keighley et al. (1979)[b]	12	Not specified	–	16/35	11/37	–	4/36	6/34	–
Cheng et al. (1981)	12	Bleeding	14/21	15/20	19/22	–	–	–	18/19
		Prolapse	4/9	10/10	5/8	–	–	–	11/11
Sim et al. (1981)	12	Bleeding	14/24	15/22	–	–	–	–	–
		Prolapse	0/7	5/7	–	–	–	–	–
Greca et al. (1981)	12	Not specified	13/33	15/28	–	–	–	–	–
Murie et al. (1982)	42	Bleeding	–	27/38	–	–	–	–	32/38
		Prolapse	–	17/25	–	–	–	–	27/29
O'Callaghan et al. (1982)	48	Not specified	–	–	–	–	65/89	–	64/88
Hancock (1982)[c]	60	1st, 2nd degree	–	–	19/22	–	–	–	–
		3rd degree	–	–	12/26	–	–	–	–
Leicester (1983)	12	Bleeding	17/35	–	–	20/38	–	–	–
		Prolapse	–	12/34	–	17/43	–	–	–
Templeton et al. (1983)	3–12	Not specified	–	33/62	–	34/60	–	–	–
Ambrose et al. (1983)	12	1st degree	–	6/17	–	8/22	–	–	–
		2nd degree	–	20/62	–	26/68	–	–	–

[a] RBL, rubber band ligation; MDA, maximal dilatation of the anus; IR, infrared coagulation; C, cryotherapy; LS, lateral sphincterotomy; H, haemorrhoidectomy.
[b] For full details of references see pp.124–125.
[c] Non-controlled trial.

Table 5.8. Haemorrhoids: Summary of results of clinical trials in Table 5.7 (at 12 months)

	Asymptomatic (% ± S.D.)		
	Injection	Rubber band ligation	Infrared coagulation
Bleeding	42 ± 28	47 ± 30	44 ± 11
Prolapse	28 ± 24	56 ± 25	38 ± 1

Thrombosed Prolapsed Haemorrhoids (strangulated piles)

A prolapsing haemorrhoid may be trapped by the anal sphincter, causing it to become swollen and irreducible. Thrombosis occurs within the internal and external haemorrhoids leading to impairment of the blood supply and eventually gangrene.

Usually all three haemorrhoids are involved but sometimes only one is affected. Although the condition commonly occurs in patients recognised to have haemorrhoids that have prolapsed in the past, this is not always the case. A proportion present for the first time with thrombosed prolapsed haemorrhoids.

Diagnosis

The history is typical, with the sudden onset of irreducible prolapse, increasing pain and swelling. An attack of diarrhoea or straining frequently precipitates the event. Inspection of the anus will confirm the diagnosis, showing circumferential thrombosis and gross oedema of the external component, with one or more internal haemorrhoids visible above often showing signs of secondary infection, ulceration and gangrene. Full examination of the rectum and anal canal should be deferred until pain has settled or examination under anaesthetic is carried out. Occasionally a carcinoma may be found and any suspicious lesion must be biopsied.

Treatment

NON-OPERATIVE TREATMENT. The natural history is of slow resolution. Pain and acute inflammatory oedema usually settle in a few days but it may take weeks for all the swelling to reduce owing to the time required for organisation of thrombosis. Non-operative treatment consists of measures to accelerate this process and to treat pain and constipation; these include bed rest, the local application of ice packs and evaporating lead lotion, analgesia and laxatives. It is almost always impossible to 'reduce' the haemorrhoids since a large part of the lesion is perianal (i.e. the thrombosed external component).

After resolution there is often surprisingly little residual abnormality and in some cases no further treatment is necessary. In others injection or rubber band ligation may be required depending on the symptoms. Some surgeons advocate an interval haemorrhoidectomy as a routine, but it is more logical to base this decision on the symptomatic outcome in the individual patient.

OPERATIVE TREATMENT. Manual dilation under general anaesthetic may dramatically improve pain, probably by relieving spasm of the sphincter. It is simple to perform and is followed by resolution of swelling over a few weeks.

Haemorrhoidectomy should be curative but is not easy to perform owing to oedema and circumferential thrombosis. There is a real danger of excising too much skin and mucosa, which may produce an anal stricture.

CHOICE OF TREATMENT. Where the acute phase is settling and there is no gangrene, conservative treatment is most appropriate. There is little to be gained by a haemorrhoidectomy at this stage since pain will be made worse and no further treatment might have been necessary after resolution. Manual dilation or haemorrhoidectomy are more suitable when pain is severe, i.e. in the early evolution of the condition. The choice depends on the preference of the surgeon. Haemorrhoidectomy should be performed only by an experienced operator.

Thrombosed Perianal Varyx (perianal haematoma)

Thrombosed perianal varyx is a very common condition. It is due to thrombosis within veins in the perianal subcutaneous plexus and it is not an extravasated haematoma. Occasionally the whole circumference of the anus may be involved, but much more usually a discrete hemispherical swelling occurs at one point at the anal verge.

Diagnosis

The patient complains of a tender anal swelling which develops over a few hours, often following exercise or straining at stool. Pain may be considerable as the clot enlarges, exciting a local inflammatory reaction, and is worse on defaecation. A tense often bluish swelling is seen at the anal verge with oedema of the overlying skin. There is no doubt on inspection and gentle palpation that the lesion is perianal and is not prolapsing from within the anal canal. Rectal digital examination and sigmoidoscopy should not be performed in the acute stage.

Treatment

As with prolapsed strangulated haemorrhoids, the lesion will resolve spontaneously. Severe pain passes in 3–4 days and usually disappears within 10 days. The swelling diminishes over a few weeks to leave a small residual fibrous nodule.

If the patient presents when pain is settling, as is often the case, local application of lead lotion, laxatives and reassurance are all that is necessary. If on the other hand the lesion is seen within the first 48–72 hours evacuation of the clot

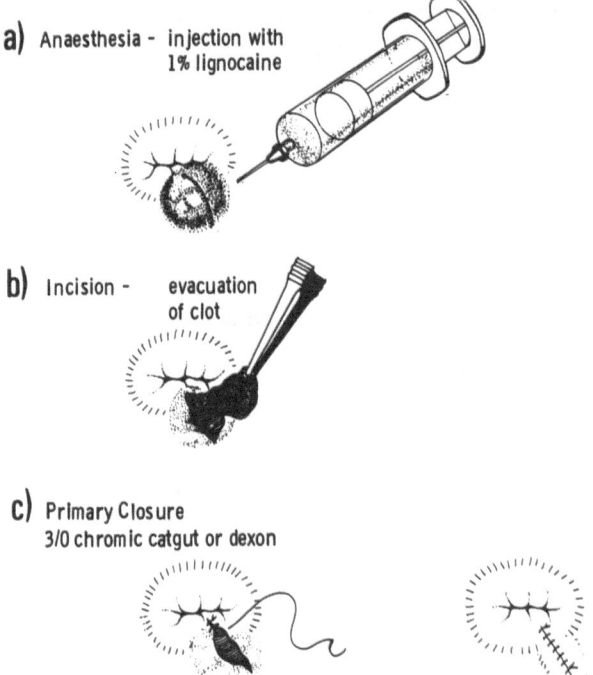

a) Anaesthesia - injection with
         1% lignocaine

b) Incision -   evacuation
                     of clot

c) Primary Closure
       3/0 chromic catgut or dexon

Fig. 5.8a–c. Excision of a thrombosed perianal varyx.

or excision gives immediate relief. Both procedures are carried out under local anaesthetic. With evacuation a skin incision over the varyx is made and the thrombus expressed. The edges are trimmed to create a flat wound which is dressed with moist gauze held in place by a T-bandage. In performing excision an elliptical incision is made, the whole lesion is removed and the wound edges closed by primary suture. Excision has the advantage that haemostasis is assured (Fig. 5.8).

Fibrous Anal Polyp

Fibrous anal polyp arises from one of the papillary processes of the dentate line. It is pedunculated and the stalk may be very long and attenuated. The lesion is composed of fibrous tissue covered by squamous epithelium.

The aetiology is unknown, but the condition is associated with chronic anal fissure and haemorrhoids. Often, however, it occurs in the absence of any other lesion.

The condition may be asymptomatic, being found on routine anorectal examination. In other cases the patient complains of a prolapsing lump often requiring digital replacement. Treatment is by excision, which should be done under anaesthesia since the lesion, being derived from the cutaneous part of the anal canal, has a sensory innervation. It is therefore not suitable for rubber band ligation.

Skin Tags

Skin tags are very common and usually are of no pathological significance. Redundancy of the perianal skin may occur in association with internal haemorrhoids, where there is a tendency for the lining of the anal canal to slide downwards. A tag may accompany an anal fissure and may be a manifestation of anal Crohn's disease, especially if it is oedematous.

Skin tags are usually asymptomatic but sometimes the patient finds their presence uncomfortable. Patients with pruritus ani are often found to have tags which in some cases, owing to difficulty in cleaning the anus after defaecation, may contribute to the condition.

The diagnosis is made on inspection. Tags can be confused with other perianal lesions, e.g. condylomata or even carcinoma, and with any prolapsing swelling. However, as they are formed by normal skin, the diagnosis should not be in doubt. If there is any doubt, removal and histological examination are indicated.

Asymptomatic tags do not need treatment. When tags are associated with a fissure, excision should be accompanied by a sphincterotomy or anal stretch. A haemorrhoidectomy is the only effective means of dealing with large symptomatic tags occurring with internal haemorrhoids.

Excision

After infiltration by local anaesthetic, the tag is excised using scissors to leave an oval wound. This should be closed by primary suture to obtain haemostasis and the wound dressed with gauze soaked in hypochlorite solution (2.5%) and held on with adhesive tape.

Anorectal Sepsis

Anorectal abscess and fistula are two phases of the same disease. About 10% of cases are associated with other pathology (Table 5.9). Anorectal sepsis varies in anatomical complexity, and its relationship to the external anal sphincter and puborectalis muscles is of the greatest importance in treatment.

Thus there are three aspects to the preoperative management: diagnosis, exclusion of other pathology and definition of the anatomical extent.

Table 5.9. Anorectal sepsis: Associated diseases

Crohn's disease
Ulcerative colitis
Hidradenitis suppurativa
Carcinoma of anus or lower rectum
Pelvic sepsis from disease of pelvic organs or intestine
Foreign bodies

Very rare:
   Tuberculosis
   Lymphogranuloma venereum
   Actinomycosis

Pathogenesis

The majority of abscesses probably originate within the intersphincteric space from infection of an anal gland. There is already a potential communication with the anal canal lumen via the anal gland duct and as the abscess expands, pus tracks to the perianal region where drainage either spontaneous or by surgical incision results in an external opening creating a fistula (Fig. 5.9). Although the anal gland–intersphincteric abscess theory is not applicable in all cases, it offers a practical basis for the classification of fistula-in-ano.

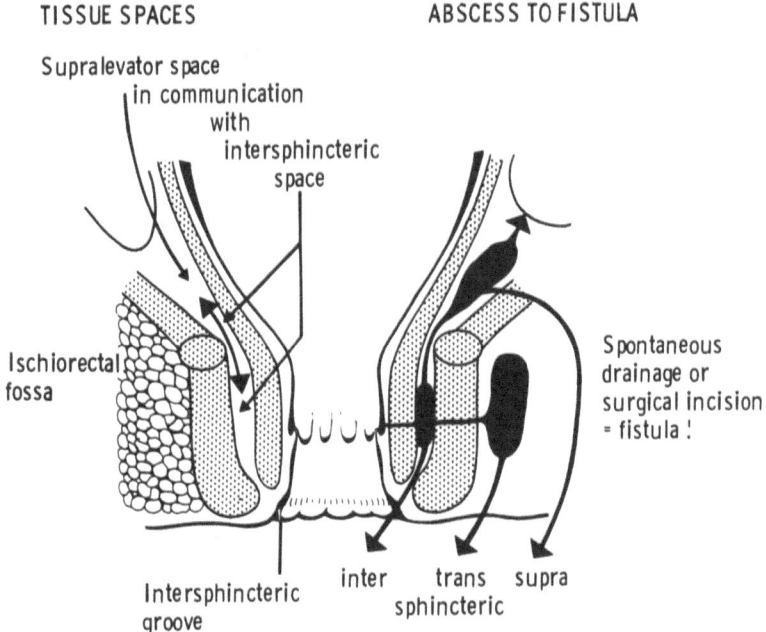

Fig. 5.9. The pathogenesis of anorectal sepsis and fistula: possible direction taken by pus spreading from an intersphincteric abscess.

Surgical Anatomy

A fistula consists of an internal opening, one or more external openings, a primary track and in many cases one or more secondary tracks. There may be chronic abscesses associated with tracks.

INTERNAL OPENING. The internal opening corresponds to the point at which the anal gland duct enters the anal canal. It is therefore most commonly located in an anal crypt. There is usually only one internal opening and the majority lie in the midline, the posterior position being more common than the anterior. In about 10% of cases of fistula it is not possible to demonstrate an internal opening even on examination under anaesthetic. In some of these the presence of scarring in a crypt suggests that an erstwhile opening has healed.

PRIMARY TRACK. The primary track connects the internal opening to the external opening. In some cases it may divide giving rise to two or more external openings. When this occurs there is often circumferential spreading of pus forming horse-shoe tracks. Circumferential extension is determined by the anatomy of the tissue spaces. Posteriorly, at least, there is no limitation to lateral tracking in the ischiorectal fossa and supralevator space and complete circumferential extension is possible in the intersphincteric space. In practice the ischiorectal fossa is the commonest site of horseshoe extension.

Fistula-in-ano can be classified according to the relationship of the primary track to the external sphincter and puborectalis (Fig. 5.10). Simple downward extension of pus in the intersphincteric space produces a perianal abscess and intersphincteric fistula (Fig. 5.10a). Penetration of the external sphincter below the puborectalis causes an ischiorectal abscess and a trans-sphincteric fistula (Fig. 5.10b). Extension of pus upwards over the puborectalis from the intersphincteric space results in a supralevator abscess which may penetrate the levator ani to enter the ischiorectal fossa and produce a suprasphincteric fistula (Fig. 5.10c). It is likely that some suprasphincteric fistulas are iatrogenic, having been caused by surgery for a simpler fistula.

Two other types of fistula occur but neither can easily be related to anal gland infection. Extrasphincteric fistulas pass directly from the rectum to the perineum lateral to the puborectalis (Fig. 5.10d). These are rare and are probably either iatrogenic, following previous fistula surgery, or due to specific disease such as Crohn's disease, carcinoma or trauma in the rectum, colon or other pelvic

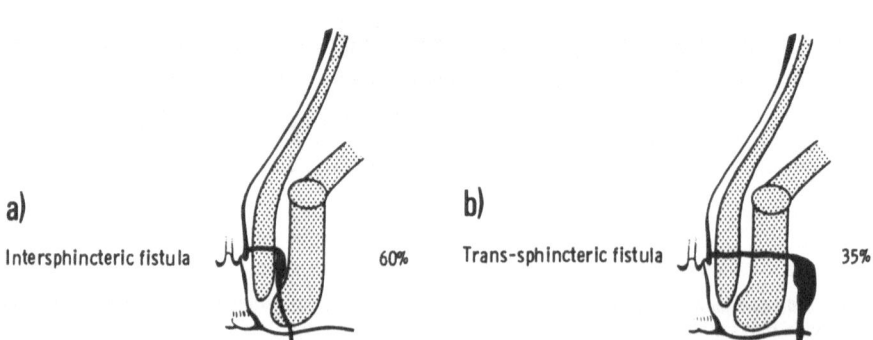

a)

Intersphincteric fistula   60%

b)

Trans-sphincteric fistula   35%

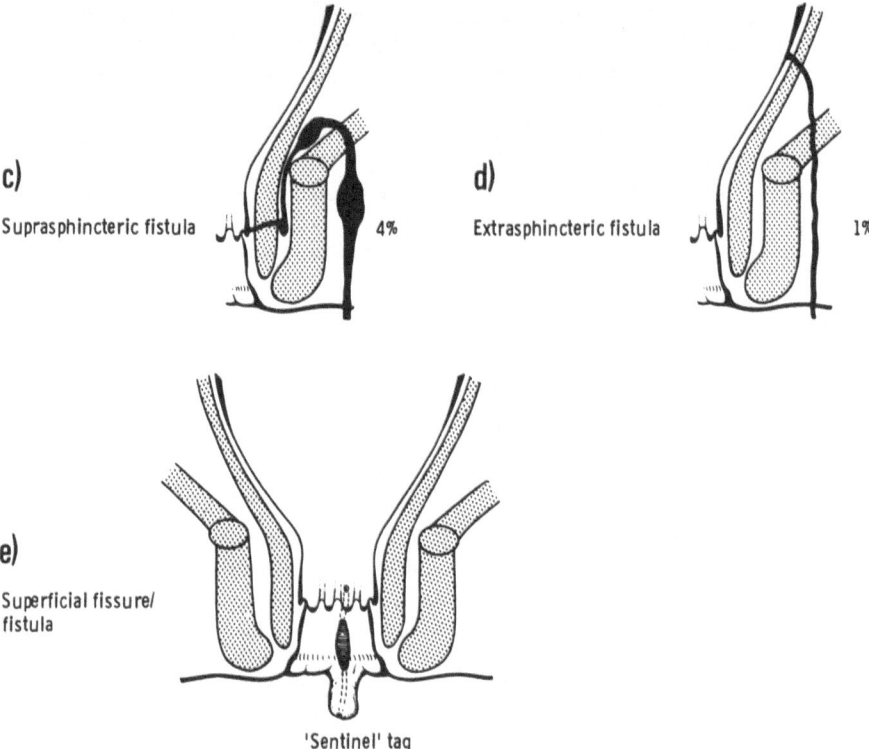

c) Suprasphincteric fistula 4%

d) Extrasphincteric fistula 1%

e) Superficial fissure/fistula

'Sentinel' tag

Fig. 5.10a–e. Classification of fistula-in-ano.

organs. Superficial fistulas are usually associated with anal fissure where undermining has led to a subcutaneous communication between the fissure and a nearby crypt (Fig. 5.10e). If superficial fistulas are excluded, 95% of fistulas-in-ano are either intersphincteric or trans-sphincteric.

Diagnosis

There are three forms of clinical presentation: acute abscess, chronic intersphincteric abscess and fistula-in-ano.

Symptoms

ACUTE ABSCESS. A patient with an acute abscess presents with pain that has increased gradually over the preceding few days, which is usually throbbing and is exacerbated by defaecation. Fever is often present and the patient may be aware of a tender perianal swelling. A discharge of pus may have been noticed.

CHRONIC INTERSPHINCTERIC ABSCESS. The history of a chronic intersphincteric abscess is characterised by periodic episodes of anal pain that resolves after a few days; the episodes may be separated by asymptomatic intervals of weeks or months.

FISTULA-IN-ANO. The cardinal symptom of a fistula-in-ano is a purulent discharge which may be constant or intermittent. Often the patient gives a history of exacerbations of pain which resolve with the discharge of pus, indicating recurrent abscess formation with spontaneous drainage. There is often a history of previous surgical drainage of an abscess or surgical attempts to treat a fistula.

Signs

ACUTE ABSCESS. With an acute abscess there are usually signs of cellulitis or of an abscess pointing in the perianal region, but sometimes these are absent if the pus is deeply placed. In the former case a digital examination per rectum is not necessary as the diagnosis is obvious, but in the latter circumstance it will be required in order to make a diagnosis. If, however, digital examination is painful, it should be stopped and arrangements made for examination under anaesthesia. An enlarged tender inguinal lymph node may be present.

CHRONIC INTERSPHINCTERIC ABSCESS. This type of abscess is a circumscribed tender lesion usually slightly smaller than a hazelnut which is most commonly located in the posterior midline. There is no external opening and the diagnosis is made on palpation, feeling the lesion between finger and thumb. Sometimes a fissure-in-ano is also present.

FISTULA-IN-ANO. External openings of a fistula-in-ano are seen on inspection of the perianal region and scars from previous surgery may also be present. The surrounding skin usually feels indurated and it may be possible to palpate the most superficial part of the primary track in its course to the internal opening. The internal opening is identified by digital palpation as an area of induration in the anal canal.

Secondary tracks and abscesses in the ischiorectal fossa and supralevator space produce induration which can be felt above the puborectalis on applying the finger downwards onto the levator plate.

Differential Diagnosis

An abscess or fistula should be distinguished from other causes of pain and associated conditions should be looked for. Other painful conditions include fissure, thrombosed external anal varyx, strangulated internal haemorrhoids, anal carcinoma, cutaneous furuncle, an infected sebaceous cyst of the perianal skin or hidradenitis suppurativa. The last three may be indistinguishable clinically from an abscess or fistula but the true diagnosis should be apparent at the time of drainage when their superficial position is revealed. A fissure does not exclude abscess or fistula, owing to their mutual association.

Occasionally a pelvic abscess may track down towards the perineum. Although this is uncommon, an intra-abdominal source should be considered when a perineal abscess is present without evidence of an internal opening in the anal canal.

Of the diseases associated with abscess or fistula Crohn's disease and hidradenitis suppurativa are the commonest. An anorectal carcinoma may invade the ischiorectal fossa to form a malignant fistula-in-ano. The diagnosis is made by feeling a mass and confirming cancer by microscopic examination of a biopsy. In all cases of anorectal sepsis sigmoidoscopy to exclude rectal disease is obligatory.

Management

Acute Abscess

The treatment of an acute abscess is by surgical drainage. With conservative management by antibiotics, the chance of success is small and delay in drainage may lead to further extension of the abscess.

Drainage is often carried out in the outpatient department, but if the abscess is extensive it is wise to admit the patient to hospital. An incision should be made at the site of maximum fluctuation or where the abscess appears to be pointing. The pus is evacuated and the cavity curetted with gentle disruption of any obvious loculi. The wound is then trimmed sufficiently to allow the insertion of a gauze dressing. Sometimes an internal opening draining pus is seen, indicating the presence of a fistula. Unless the surgeon is confident that such a track is well below the puborectalis it is wiser in the acute stage not to lay it open since it may not be possible to be certain of the relationship of the fistula to the anal sphincter. A culture of enteric organisms from the original pus usually indicates true anorectal sepsis with the likelihood of a fistula being present. A growth of cutaneous organisms (e.g. *Staphylococcus aureus*) suggests that the original abscess was a perianal furuncle and therefore not likely to be associated with fistula.

The cavity is dressed with gauze soaked in saline or hypochlorite solution and held on by a T-bandage. Dressings are changed at 24–48 hours, after the patient has soaked the wound in a bath. Thereafter, the regime consists of twice-daily baths and redressings. Dressings should be tucked into the wound simply to keep the edges apart to prevent bridging and pocketing. Packing the wound with ribbon gauze is uncomfortable and delays healing.

It is good practice to re-examine the patient under anaesthetic 7–10 days later when healing can be assessed and any fistula identified and laid open.

Chronic Intersphincteric Abscess

The treatment of a chronic intersphincteric abscess is by surgical excision of the entire abscess; it therefore involves division of the internal sphincter up to the most proximal extent of the abscess and division of the lower part of the external sphincter to ensure as flat a wound as possible. The wound is left open and dressed in the same manner as that left after treating an acute abscess. It usually heals in 2–3 weeks but healing may take longer and the patient should be warned of this.

Fistula-in-Ano

The principles of operative treatment for a fistula-in-ano are to lay open the primary track, drain secondary tracks and abscesses and create a wound which will allow easy dressing.

These principles must be applied without risking continence, which will be maintained if the puborectalis and upper external anal sphincter are preserved. In patients with normal muscles, division of the lower internal and external sphincters does not cause faecal incontinence (although sometimes difficulty in holding flatus occurs), but in those with a weak pelvic floor continence may be threatened.

PREOPERATIVE ASSESSMENT (Table 5.10). It is therefore essential to define the anatomy of a fistula before treatment, the key being the site of the primary track and its relationship to the puborectalis. In addition the presence of secondary tracks or abscesses should be established since treatment will fail if they are not drained.

The preoperative assessment should be made in the unanaesthetised patient so that the puborectalis, which marks the anorectal junction, can be felt on voluntary contraction.

Table 5.10. Fistula-in-ano: Assessment

Perineum	Inspection	External openings (number and sites)
		? Abscess (reddening and swelling)
	Palpation	Direction of tracks (perianal induration)
Anal canal	Rectal digital examination	*Primary track*
		Internal opening (induration)
		Site
		Relationship to puborectalis
		?*Secondary tracks* (supralevator induration)
Rectum	Sigmoidoscopy ± radiology	Proctitis
		Carcinoma
		Diverticular disease
		Disease of other pelvic organs

Primary Track (Fig. 5.11). The internal opening which marks the point of entry of the primary track into the anal canal is felt as a localised area of induration, most commonly in the midline. Once it has been identified the patient should be asked to contract the pelvic floor; this will allow the puborectalis to be felt. An estimation of the amount of sphincter between the puborectalis and the internal opening can then be made (Fig. 5.12). Only occasionally will there be so little sphincter that a simple laying open will risk continence. Experience is needed to make this judgement, but if laying open is considered too hazardous the operation can be modified, for example by using a seton suture.

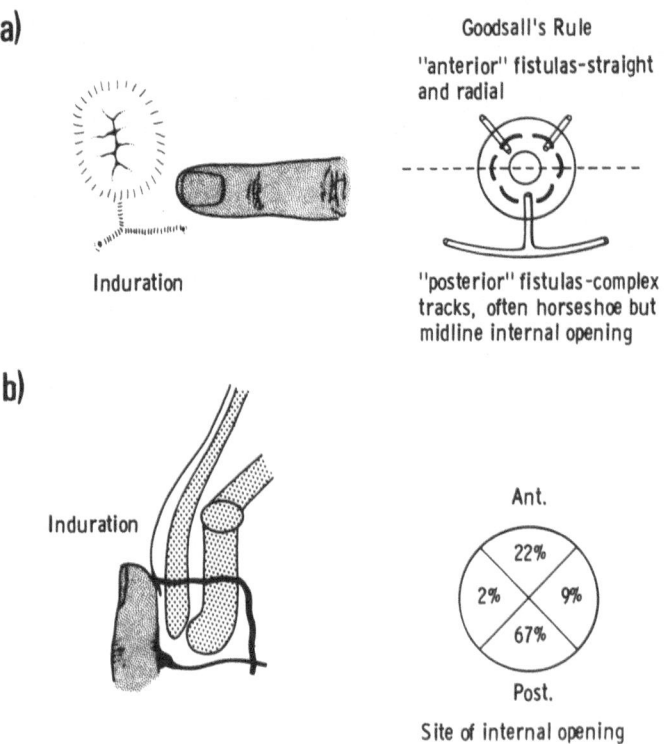

Fig. 5.11a, b. Identification of the primary track.

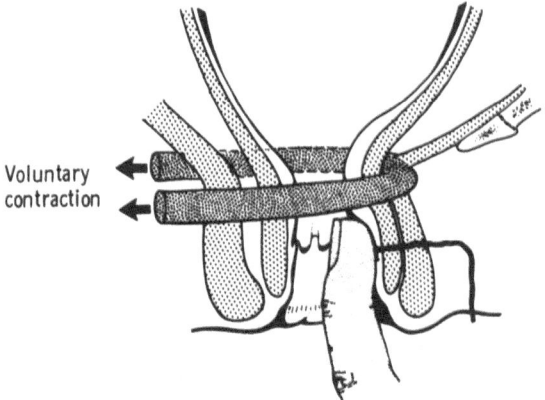

Fig. 5.12. Assessment of the relationship of the primary track to the puborectalis.

Except in the rare situation of a suprasphincteric fistula, definition of the course of the primary track to the perineum is less important than location of the internal opening. However, the track can sometimes be palpated as a core of induration in the perianal region and its likely direction may also be guessed by applying Goodsall's rule. This states that fistulas with an external opening in relation to the anterior half of the anus tend to pass radially to the internal opening. Where an external opening is related to the posterior half of the anus, the track is usually circumferential, passing towards an internal opening in the posterior midline.

Secondary Tracks and Abscesses (Fig. 5.13). Secondary tracks are identified by the presence of induration away from the primary track. In practice this is most likely to cause supralevator induration felt on digital examination. Fig. 5.13 shows examples of secondary extension above the puborectalis. In Fig. 5.13a pus from an intersphincteric fistula has extended directly upwards into the supra-levator space, with no breach of the external sphincter fistula where an upward

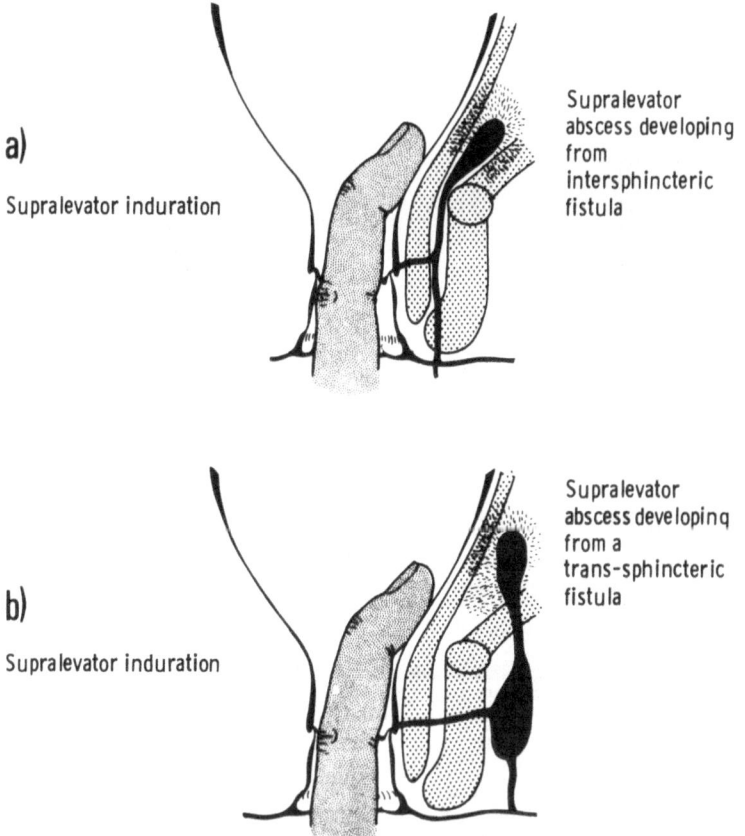

a)

Supralevator induration

Supralevator abscess developing from intersphincteric fistula

b)

Supralevator induration

Supralevator abscess developing from a trans-sphincteric fistula

Fig. 5.13a, b. Assessment of secondary tracks and abscesses.

extension through the apex of the ischiorectal fossa has occurred. In both cases inflammation in the region of the levator ani will be palpable as induration above the anorectal ring. On finding supralevator induration the surgeon knows that simple laying open of the primary track will be inadequate and that secondary extension must be present.

The reader is referred to textbooks of surgery for a detailed account of the operative treatment of the various forms of anal fistula.

Anal Crohn's Disease

Anal lesions are the first manifestation of large bowel Crohn's disease in 25% of cases and overall occur in 50%–70% of patients with colonic or rectal involvement. Their incidence in small bowel or ileocaecal Crohn's disease without apparent colonic disease is 10%–30%. The type and relative frequency of lesions are shown in Table 5.11. Presentation may be acute or chronic depending on the lesion, and anal disease may be the most troublesome aspect for the patient or it may be overshadowed by symptoms from other sites of involvement.

Table 5.11. Crohn's disease: Anal lesions at presentation[a]

Fissure	59
Fistula/abscess	34
Oedematous tags	22
Ulceration	12
Skin oedema	9
Rectovaginal fistula	4
Bluish discoloration	2

[a] In 127 of 251 new patients at St. Mark's Hospital, London, 1979–83.

Diagnosis

Anal Crohn's disease is more likely if any of the following perineal features are present:

Multiple anal lesions

Oedematous skin tags

Blue-crimson coloration of the skin

Involvement of the labia or groins

Indolent ulceration

Extensive anorectal sepsis

High fistulation (including rectovaginal fistulas)

There may be other symptoms of Crohn's disease due to colitis or small bowel disease and general symptoms of weight loss or anorexia.

General and abdominal signs of Crohn's disease may be found and sigmoidoscopy is likely to show abnormalities, the most common of which is patchy inflammation. A rectal biopsy should be taken and radiological examination of the small and large bowel carried out. Granulomatoma are found in about 75% of rectal biopsy specimens although they occur much less frequently in tissue taken from the anal lesion itself (33%).

Management

The aim of management should be to relieve symptoms with the minimum procedure possible.

Fissure

Sphincterotomy for fissure runs the risk of creating a perianal wound which may fail to heal and lead to suppuration. An anal stretch avoiding an incision may be preferable, although this must be gentle to avoid sphincter damage.

Abscess

Anorectal abscesses should be treated by surgical drainage. With a supralevator abscess extensive local surgery may be necessary.

Fistula

Most anal fistulas in Crohn's disease have an internal opening well below the puborectalis. Low fistulas of this type comprise two-thirds of cases, a proportion only slightly less than is observed among patients with non-Crohn's fistulas (73%). Conventional laying open of low fistulas in Crohn's disease results in healing in 90% of cases, and this is therefore the treatment of choice. Healing of high fistulas after laying open occurs in only about 50% of cases and surgery should therefore involve either laying open or more simply the drainage of abscesses to relieve pain and acute inflammation depending on assessment of the individual case. In the latter circumstance the patient often tolerates a persistent small discharge of pus and is able to lead a normal life despite it. Some may be helped by additional treatment with cotrimoxazole and metronidazole, which often reduce discharge although rarely promote permanent healing.

There is some evidence that resection of coexisting intestinal disease may be followed by healing of an anal fistula. If so the chance appears to be greater in cases with small bowel rather than large bowel involvement. Severe anorectal sepsis uncontrolled by local surgery is an indication for proctocolectomy. In practice this is necessary only in a small proportion of patients with fistula

(10%–15%), most of whom also have severe rectal disease as a contributory factor. Thus the majority of cases can be successfully managed by local surgery, which may, however, need to be repeated.

Haemorrhoids

Treatment of haemorrhoids in patients with Crohn's disease has a high incidence of complications (50%). Haemorrhoidectomy in particular may leave the patient with chronic unhealing anal wounds or fistula-in-ano (67%) which may necessitate excision of the rectum. Surgery for haemorrhoids is therefore contraindicated in Crohn's disease.

Ulceration and Wounds

Gauze soaked in hypochlorite solution or prednisolone is the most suitable wound dressing. Regular baths and irrigation of the wound with saline are advised if there is much pus. Surgery to lay open undermining sinuses or to remove tags may be necessary.

Stenosis

An anal or rectal stenosis can usually be managed by dilatation using the finger or graded Hegar's dilators. Only rarely is rectal excision required.

Hidradenitis Suppurativa

Hidradenitis suppurativa is a fairly common condition which may be mistaken for fistula-in-ano. It is due to infection of apocrine skin glands, which are glands found in the axillae, groins, external genitalia, nape of the neck and areola of the nipples as well as in the perianal region. Anal lesions occur in about one-third of patients with hidradenitis. The disease predominantly affects young adults and does not appear until the glands begin to function after puberty. The sex ratio of cases is approximately equal although perianal involvement may be more common in males. There is an association with acne.

The cause is unknown, but it is likely that there is an abnormality in the material secreted by the glands. Retention of secretion results in stasis and infection leading to abscess formation. The glands are deeply placed in the dermis and suppuration may extend into the subcutaneous tissues forming tracks or large areas of undermining lined by granulation tissue (Fig. 5.14). Subcutaneous extension may break through to the surface as sinuses some distance from the original lesion. This infective process is accompanied by attempts at repair, with fibrosis in the skin and subcutaneous tissue.

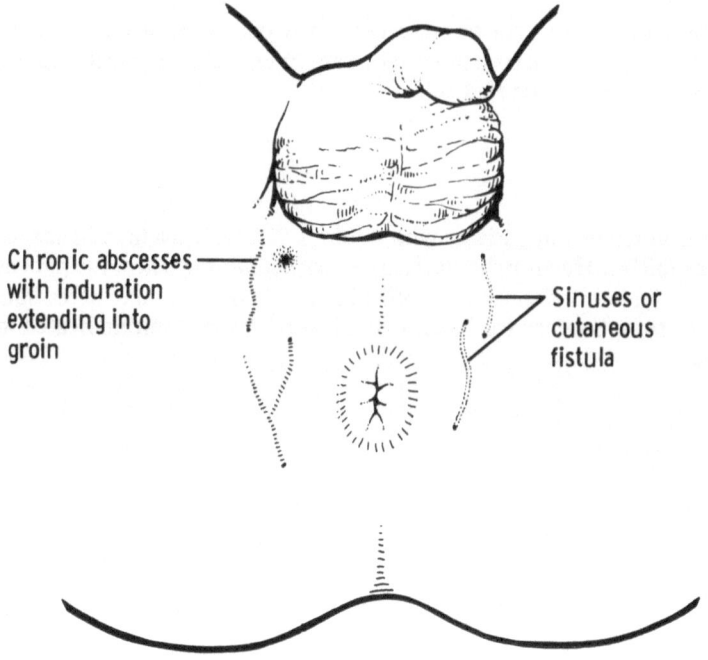

Chronic abscesses
with induration
extending into
groin

Sinuses or
cutaneous
fistula

Fig. 5.14. Hidradenitis suppurativa.

Diagnosis

Symptoms

An acute lesion begins as a localised tender nodule around an apocrine gland
which gradually resolves over a few days with or without a small discharge of
pus. There may then be recurrent exacerbations at the same site, while other
lesions may form. Discharge from sinuses is intermittent, producing relief of pain
when it occurs. It is usually thin, though purulent, and has an unpleasant odour.

Signs

On inspecting the perianal region localised nodules a few millimetres in diameter
will be seen. In severe cases, obvious thickening and oedema of the surrounding
skin and induration along subcutaneous tracks will be evident. Frequently one
sinus opening will communicate with another, forming a subcutaneous fistula.

Other sites liable to be affected should be inspected and a full anorectal
examination is also important since there is an association between hidradenitis
and fistula-in-ano and possibly also with squamous cell carcinoma of the perianal
skin.

Differential Diagnosis

The disease may be confused with furunculosis, an infected sebaceous cyst, acute perianal abscess or with the external opening of a fistula-in-ano, but the typical appearance of the lesions and their frequent presence in other sites will confirm the diagnosis.

Management

The treatment is surgical. A localised abscess should be incised and the granulation tissue in the cavity curetted. Subcutaneous tracks and fistulas should be laid open and curetted and the wounds left to heal by secondary intention. Occasionally, where there is extensive involvement of a given area, wide local excision is necessary. Large open wounds heal slowly by secondary intention and healing may be accelerated by skin grafting.

Incision and laying open is repeated as new lesions develop. Unfortunately there is no effective prophylaxis at present.

Sexually Transmitted Diseases

The prevalence of sexually transmitted disease is rising and has become an epidemic problem on a huge scale. Syphilis is now more common than it was 10 years ago and it has been estimated that throughout the world over 200 million people become infected with gonorrhoea annually. As if this were not enough, non-specific genital infection is commoner still and it appears that at least 50% of these cases are due to infection with *Chlamydia trachomatis.*

Diagnosis

It is certain that patients with sexually transmitted diseases will be seen in the rectal clinic; the problem is to identify them. Anal lesions are produced by many such diseases including syphilis (primary chancre, condylomata lata), condylomata acuminata (warts), AIDS, herpes simplex, molluscum contageosum, perianal fungal infection and rare diseases such as chancroid and granuloma inguinale. Others, for example gonorrhoea and non-specific genital infection, cause proctitis without external manifestations. Gonorrhoea in females is frequently asymptomatic. Prevalence is three to four times higher in large cities than in rural areas. Male patients are often homosexual.

Although common, sexually transmitted disease will be missed if the diagnosis is not considered. Any anal cutaneous lesion should arouse suspicion, as a primary syphilitic chancre may resemble a simple fissure, external haemorrhoids, lesions in Crohn's diease or anal carcinoma.

The genitalia should always be examined and it is preferable to request serological and bacteriological tests when in doubt. These should be routine in diseases such as condylomata acuminata which are known to be transmitted by genital contact.

Management

Management involves treating the patient and tracing possible contacts. A patient diagnosed as having a sexually transmitted disease must be referred to a specialist dealing with these conditions. The proctologist may, however, help by establishing some of the patient's contacts and making clear to the patient the diagnosis and the need to avoid sexual intercourse while in an infectious state.

Syphilis

Syphilis is caused by the organism *Treponema pallidum* and is transmitted by direct physical contact. In Western society 50% of cases are male homosexuals, infection usually occurring by anal intercourse. The primary chancre is the first manifestation of the disease and appears about 4–5 weeks after exposure. It forms at the site of contact, which is usually at the anal verge, anal canal, vulva or glans penis, and appears as a raised circular indurated lesion measuring about 1 cm across. It may discharge and be painful, but heals spontaneously after 2 weeks or so. The inguinal nodes are enlarged during this stage.

Some weeks later the secondary stage appears. This is a systemic disturbance with fever, malaise, lymphadenopathy, arthropathy and generalised cutaneous eruptions which can mimic many other skin diseases. It resolves after a few weeks. During this stage, condylomata lata are seen around the anus. These are multiple lesions with a slightly elevated edge and flat surface, producing an exudate rich in treponemes. Tertiary syphilis with involvement of the nervous and vascular systems and the formation of gummata develops some years later.

The diagnosis can be made by dark-ground microscopical examination of exudate from the primary chancre or condylomata lata to identify *Treponema pallidum*. Of the serological tests listed in Table 5.12 the VDRL is most used. It is quite possible that the patient will also be infected with gonorrhoeae, and swabs from the urethra, vagina and rectum should be sent for examination.

Gonorrhoea

Gonorrhoea is a common disease caused by the organism *Neisseria gonorrhoeae* which infects the mucous membranes of the vagina, urethra, rectum and oropharynx. About one-third of cases are homosexual males. The incubation period is from 2 to 10 days. Anorectal infection results from anal intercourse in both sexes, but in females it is said that the rectum may also become involved by infection spreading from the genital tract. In half the cases anorectal gonorrhoea

Table 5.12. Syphilis: Tests

Test	Material from patient	Type	Positivity	Comments
Venereal Disease Research Laboratory slide test (VDRL)[a]	Serum	Flocculation	Early ($\geqslant$ 2 weeks)	Non-specific, cheap
Treponema pallidum haemagglutination test (TPHA)[a]	Serum	Haemagglutination	Late (several weeks) primary syphilis positive in 50%–70% secondary syphilis positive in 90 + %	Specific, cheap
Fluorescent *Treponema*-antibody test (FTA)	Serum	Indirect immunofluorescence	Early ($\geqslant$ 2 weeks)	Specific, sensitive, expensive
Dark-ground microscopy	Exudate from lesions (live treponemes)	Direct identification of treponeme	Immediate	
Cardiolipin Wassermann test } *Treponema pallidum* immobilisation test (TPI) }	No longer used			

[a] Tests used in initial screening.

produces no symptoms; when symptoms are present these are usually an anal discharge with perianal discomfort. There are usually no external signs but proctoscopy shows abnormal features. The mucosa is oedematous and often coated by pus. There is no marked injection as seen in ulcerative colitis or Crohn's disease and ulceration is very rare. The changes usually involve the lower rectum although they may occasionally extend into the distal sigmoid colon. The diagnosis is made by isolating the organisms from swabs taken from the urethra, vagina or rectum. These should be placed immediately into a suitable transport medium (e.g. Stewart's medium) and plated as soon as possible.

Non-specific Genital Infection

One of the greatest advances in genitourinary medicine in recent years has been the recognition that many cases of non-specific genital infection are caused by *Chlamydia trachomatis*. This is a member of the trachoma-psittacosis group of organisms. Improved culture techniques have enabled isolation of the organism (if looked for carefully), and if several swabs are taken for examination positive cultures are obtained in over 50% of patients with non-specific genital infection.

The clinical features and course are very similar to those of gonorrhoea. Thus urethritis, vaginitis and proctitis occur, the last being the result of infection during anal intercourse. Proctitis may cause a discharge with anal irritation and the sigmoidoscopic findings are similar to those of gonorrhoeal proctitis, with, in addition, the presence of small follicular nodules on the rectal mucosa. Sometimes the eyes (conjunctivitis, keratitis) and joints (Reiter's disease) may be affected. Again, swabs from the rectum, urethra and vagina should be taken to identify the organism.

Condylomata Acuminata (anal warts)

Condylomata acuminata are very common and are caused by an antigenic variant of the papilloma virus that is responsible for cutaneous warts. Transmission is by direct contact and over 50% of patients are homosexual males.

Diagnosis

SYMPTOMS. The patient may notice the swelling himself but more often complains of irritation and discharge, sometimes with blood on the toilet paper after wiping. Difficulty in maintaining anal hygiene is responsible for an unpleasant smell due to faecal soiling and to malodorous discharge.

SIGNS. The warts usually measure a few millimetres across but may vary from minute pinhead lesions to 1-2 cm in diameter. Small lesions are sessile and hemispherical but as they enlarge they become pendunculated and develop a finely serrated surface. They are usually multiple and sometimes cover the anus and perianal region in a carpet-like manner. Extension onto the labia, scrotum and groin may occur and the penis is often involved. In about 50% of cases they encroach into the anal canal and in about 10% the lower rectum is affected. There is a tendency for spontaneous involution and lesions in this phase have a smooth surface often surmounted by a dark punctum. Condylomata acuminata are premalignant and in about 2% of cases a frank squamous cell carcinoma is found.

It is essential to exclude other sexually transmitted diseases, particularly syphilis and gonorrhoea. Serological tests should be carried out and a rectal swab taken at proctoscopy if there is any suspicion of gonococcal proctitis.

Condylomata acuminata may be confused with anal skin tags, condylomata lata of secondary syphilis and squamous cell carcinoma. If there is any doubt, examination of exudate under dark-ground illumination and histological examination of biopsy material is necessary.

Management

The disease can be treated by the local application of podophyllin in spirit (25%), injection of cytotoxic agents (e.g. bleomycin) directly into the lesions, or by surgical destruction or excision. Podophyllin is suitable if few warts are present. It is irritant to skin and should therefore be carefully applied to the lesions alone and must never be used where open wounds or fissuring are present. Two applications per week using a pledget of gauze mounted on an orange stick are continued until the warts have disappeared. This treatment is unsuitable where the anal canal and rectum are involved. It has the further disadvantage that regular and frequent outpatient visits are required. Injection of bleomycin into the lesions has been claimed to be successful in about 70% of cases.

Surgical treatment is necessary if the warts are extensive, particularly when the anal canal is involved. Destruction can be effected by diathermy fulguration or by cryotherapy. Both methods cause damage to the surrounding normal skin with pain, discharge and often delayed healing. Scissor excision of the warts leaves a clean wound without damaged edges and thus avoids these drawbacks (Fig. 5.15). Postoperative pain is usually slight and healing rapid, occurring in only a few days. The excision is facilitated by the subcutaneous injection of a solution of physiological saline containing adrenaline in a dilution of 1:200 000. This tends to separate the lesions as the skin is stretched by the injection, making accurate excision easier; the adrenaline acts as a haemostatic agent. The surgical treatment of warts permits removal of lesions in the anal canal and rectum, not possible with podophyllin.

About 60% of patients are cured by scissor excision after one treatment and a further 30% by two. Three or more treatments are required in the remaining 10%.

Acquired Immunodeficiency Syndrome (AIDS)

In 1981 the Centers for Disease Control in the USA reported an acquired immune deficiency syndrome in apparently previously healthy homosexual males, who presented with severe opportunistic infections, Kaposi's sarcoma and lymphatic

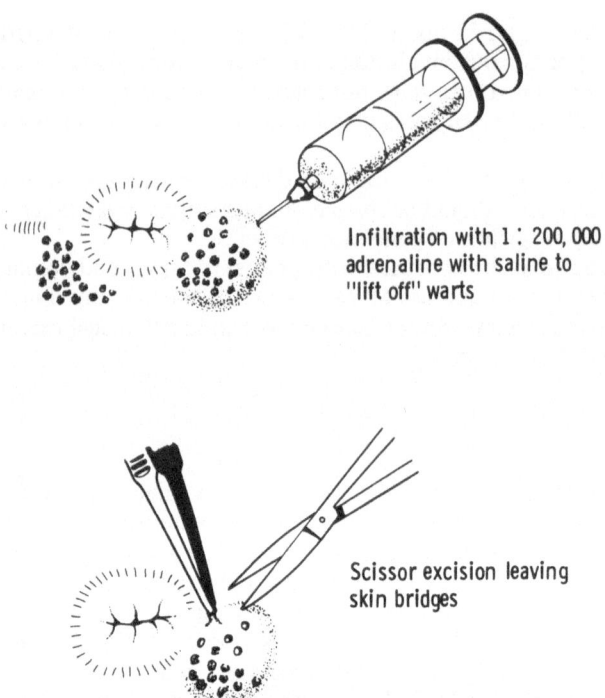

Infiltration with 1 : 200, 000
adrenaline with saline to
"lift off" warts

Scissor excision leaving
skin bridges

Fig. 5.15. Scissor excision of condylomata acuminata (anal warts).

malignancies. By August 1983 over 2000 cases had been reported in the USA and 20 other countries, with an intermediate mortality of 40% but probably approaching 100% in time.

Recent studies suggest that the disease is caused by infection with a variant of human T-lymphotrophic virus (HTLV-III) with a low-grade infectivity similar to that of hepatitis B. The incubation period is believed to be of the order of a year. Infection causes severe suppression of cell-mediated immunity leading to infection by opportunist organisms. Major risk groups have been identified and include homosexual males, intravenous drug abusers, haemophiliacs, Haitians (who probably have had homosexual contact) and females and children who have been in close contact with patients with AIDS (Table 5.13). Transmission of the virus by contaminated blood transfusion has now been reported.

Some opportunist organisms found in patients with AIDS are shown in Table 5.14. The commonest is *Pneumocystis carinii*, but the patient may develop overwhelming infection with cytomegalovirus, *Candida*, herpes simplex (hominis), toxoplasma and *Cryptococcus neoformans*. Bowel infection with *Entamoeba histolytica, Giardia lamblia, Shigella, Salmonella* and *Campylobacter* is common. A number of patients have presented with chronic unexplained lymphadenopathy and it may be that this represents a prodromal illness of the full AIDS syndrome. About a third of patients develop Kaposi's sarcoma.

Table 5.13. AIDS: Predisposition[a]

	Cases	
	No.	%
Homosexual or bisexual[b]	1427	71
Intravenous drug abuse	339	17
Haitian	105	5
Haemophiliac	15	1
No apparent predisposition	122	6

[a] Data from the National Institute of Health, August 1983.
[b] All males.

Table 5.14. AIDS: Opportunistic infecting organisms[a]

Infecting organism	No. of cases
Cytomegalovirus	31
Candida	29
Pneumocystis carinii	26
Mycobacterium avium intracellulare	15
Cryptococcus neoformans	8
Herpes simplex (hominis)	7
Cryptosporidiosis	5
Toxoplasma gondii	5
Herpes zoster	4

[a] Data from the National Institute of Health, August 1983. Infections in 53 patients at the NIH, Bethesda, Maryland.

The disease may present as pneumonia, enteritis, generalised lymphadeno-pathy, encephalopathy and herpes infection. Often recurrent herpes produces extensive genital and perianal ulceration and AIDS may therefore be seen in the rectal clinic. These lesions may be mistaken for cutaneous Crohn's disease.

If the diagnosis is suspected on clinical grounds the patient should be admitted and a blood specimen sent for tests of lymphocyte function. Profound lympho-paenia is characteristic and appropriate monoclonal antibody reactions demon-strate a reduction in the helper/inducer T lymphocyte population. An immunolo-gical test is now available to detect the presence of antibody to the HLV-III virus.

Further investigation is aimed at identifying an opportunist infecting organism from throat swabs, blood, urine, stool, cutaneous ulcers, etc.

There is no known cure for AIDS and no patient seen so far has regained immunological competence. Treatment is directed against opportunist infection.

Herpes Simplex

Herpes simplex is caused by the virus herpes hominis Type 2. It is transmitted by direct sexual contact and causes lesions on the penis and in the anorectal area. The incubation period varies from 5 to 25 days and the first symptom is pain.

This can be very severe and is followed 2–3 days later by the appearance of small bullous lesions. At this stage the pain is replaced by soreness and irritation. The lesions then crust and heal spontaneously. Ulceration of bullae may be followed by secondary infection with inguinal lymphadenopathy. Spontaneous relapses may occur.

The diagnosis is made on the clinical picture and on demonstrating a typical cytopathic effect in tissue culture. Other coexisting sexually transmitted diseases must be excluded.

As yet there is no specific treatment for herpes simplex. Local steroids and idoxuridine are ineffective but acyclovir (Zovirax) has been reported to be of use particularly for a first attack of the disease. Symptomatic treatment including analgesics and local dressings should be carried out.

Molluscum Contageosum

Molluscum contageosum, caused by a virus of the pox group, is transmitted by direct physical contact anywhere in the body including the genital organs and perineum. The incubation period is 3–6 weeks and the lesion itself appears as a flattened round vesicle measuring 3 mm in diameter with an umbilicated centre. There is no pain and the chief importance of the disease is that it is an indication of more serious sexually transmitted diseases. The lesions are readily destroyed with undiluted phenol applied individually to each.

Lymphogranuloma Venereum

Lymphogranuloma venereum is a rare condition and is caused by a member of the genus *Chlamydia*. After an incubation period of 1–4 weeks a small vesicular lesion appears. The lesion rapidly disappears but there follows enlargement of the inguinal nodes. This progresses to form an indurated mass of lymph nodes in the groins often with erythema of the overlying skin. There may be an influenza-like illness with malaise, anorexia, fever, headache and joint pains. The disease varies according to the site of the initial inoculation. Infection of the rectum produces a proctitis sometimes leading to fistulation or stricture, and pelvic pain from intra-abdominal lymph node enlargement may occur. Chronic inflammation damages lymphatics resulting in lymphoedema.

The diagnosis is made from the history and clinical finding and is confirmed by a complement fixation test. Treatment is by tetracycline given for 14 days. All sexual partners should be examined and treated if necessary.

Chancroid and Granuloma Inguinale

Chancroid and granuloma inguinale are rarely seen in Europe. Chancroid is caused by *Haemophilus ducreyi*, and results in multiple ulcers and abscesses which may affect the perineum. The condition may be confused with herpes infection and the diagnosis is made by culture of the organism. Treatment is with tetracycline and sulphonamides.

Granuloma inguinale is caused by *Calymmatobacterium granulomatis*, a Gram-negative bacillus that produces chronic granulomatous infection around the site of inoculation. The condition presents as a red, hard, shining mass around the anus or on the genitalia. Diagnosis is confirmed by biopsy and high doses of tetracycline or streptomycin are usually effective.

Malignant Anal Tumours

Malignant tumours of the anus account for only 3%–4% of large bowel tumours. They are classified by histological type into:

Squamous cell
Basaloid (cloacogenic)
Adenocarcinoma
Basal cell carcinoma
Malignant melanoma

Over 60% of cases are of squamous cell type and 20%–30% are basaloid. The other types are rare.

Squamous cell carcinoma arises from the cutaneous part of the anal canal or from the perianal skin and basaloid carcinoma from the transitional zone. There is a higher prevalence in homosexuals and some cases occur in pre-existing condylomata acuminata or Bowen's disease.

Patients can be divided into those with true anal canal carcinoma (70%) and those with carcinoma of the anal margin (30%).

Squamous Cell and Basaloid Carcinoma of the Anal Canal

Anal canal carcinoma is more common in females. The tumour may grow upwards to the rectum or downwards to the anal margin and also tends to penetrate the sphincter to invade the ischiorectal fossa and pelvic floor. Metastases to retrorectal or inguinal lymph nodes occur depending on the level of the primary tumour.

Diagnosis

SYMPTOMS. Symptoms include the awareness of a mass, pain, offensive odour, bleeding, difficulty in defaecation, the passage of thin stools and faecal incontinence. A groin lump may be noticed and general symptoms of dissemination may be present.

SIGNS. There is a mass or ulcer in the anal canal which is often tender. Inguinal lymphadenopathy may be present, and enlarged nodes mobile or fixed. The diagnosis is confirmed by biopsy, for which a general anaesthetic may be needed. CLINICAL STAGE. Dissemination to the liver and lungs is assessed by liver scan and chest X-ray; computerised tomography of the pelvis to determine local spread is indicated where the tumour is large.

The TNM classification of local clinical staging given in Table 5.15 can be directly related to survival and also influences the choice of treatment.

Table 5.15. Anal carcinoma: TNM clinical staging. Definition of T stage

Anal canal carcinoma

T1	Less than one-third of circumference or length of anal canal involved. No infiltration of external sphincter
T2	More than one-third of circumference or length of anal canal involved, or infiltration of external sphincter
T3	Extension to rectum or skin
T4	Invasion of other structures

Anal margin carcinoma

T1	Less than 2 cm in diameter. No deep infiltration of dermis
T2	2-5 cm in diameter. Superficial infiltration of dermis
T3	More than 5 cm in diameter or infiltration through dermis
T4	Invasion of muscle or bone

Treatment

Since the disease is uncommon there have been no controlled clinical trials comparing various treatments. Squamous cell carcinoma and basaloid carcinoma are sensitive to radiotherapy, which offers an attractive alternative where total rectal excision would otherwise be necessary. As expected the effectiveness of either treatment modality depends on the stage of the tumour. For T1 and T2 stage growths radiotherapy (given either by external beam (60–70 Gy) or by fractionated interstitial radium (50–60 Gy)) and total rectal excision will produce similar 5-year survival rates of about 60% overall. This falls to 20%–30% for T3 and T4 tumours or where lymph nodes are involved. There is a fairly high incidence of failure to obtain local control by radiotherapy (about 20%–30%) and severe radionecrosis has been reported in 5%–35% of cases, being more likely after external beam treatment. Up to 75% of patients have some impairment of anal sphincter function after radiotherapy. Major surgery has an operative mortality of 5%–10% and produces similar 5-year survival rates to radiotherapy. Pelvic recurrence occurs in 15%–50% of patients after total rectal excision. A small group of selected patients with T1 lesions (approximately 5%–10% of cases) may be suitable for local excision, for which the 5-year survival rate is 60%–85%.

Recently a multidisciplinary approach has been used in which patients are treated preoperatively with external beam irradiation (30 Gy) and chemotherapy (5-fluorouracil, mitomycin C) over 3 weeks before abdominoperineal excision.

Examination of the operative specimen has failed to show residual tumour in a high proportion of cases (45%–55%) and more recently simple wide local excision biopsy of the tumour area has been employed if there is no clinical evidence of persistent growth. Where no residual tumour is found in the biopsy, no further surgery is undertaken.

Squamous Cell Carcinoma of the Anal Margin

Squamous cell carcinoma of the anal margin is more common in males and behaves in a similar fashion to skin squamous carcinoma elsewhere. It has a greater tendency to spread to inguinal nodes than anal canal carcinoma. It can also be staged by the TNM system (Table 5.15). Treatment is by radiotherapy or surgical local excision, results for the two methods being similar (50%–70% 5-year survival). Salvage surgery is necessary where radiotherapy used as primary treatment does not achieve local control.

Squamous Cell Carcinoma Involving Inguinal Lymph Nodes

Patients who present with involved inguinal lymph nodes have a very low prospect of cure (10% 5-year survival). However, those who develop lymphadenopathy after primary treatment can be salvaged by treatment with a prospect of 5-year survival in 30%–40% of cases. Prophylactic treatment of nodes apparently uninvolved at initial presentation does not improve survival. If nodes are mobile, block dissection or radiotherapy is indicated. Radiotherapy should be used if they are fixed. Monthly follow-up for at least 6 months is advised for detection of any developing lymphadenopathy after primary treatment of any anal carcinoma.

Adenocarcinoma

A low rectal cancer may invade the anal canal and should be treated by total rectal excision. Involvement of the anal skin, however, may result in spread to inguinal glands. Rarely adenocarcinoma develops in the anal canal as a primary, possibly from anal gland or transitional epithelium; it may also arise in a long-standing anal fistula.

Basal Cell Carcinoma

Basal cell cancer of the anal skin is rare. It usually forms an irregular ulcer with hard raised edges. Treatment is by local excision but radiotherapy is equally effective. The inguinal glands are never involved and the prognosis is good.

Malignant Melanoma

Anal malignant melanoma is fortunately rare since it metastasises rapidly and very few patients survive more than 3 years after diagnosis. The lesion usually presents as an anal nodule and owing to its bluish-black colour it may be confused with a thrombosed haemorrhoid or perianal varyx. Often the tumour is quite large on presentation, although there may be few symptoms. The diagnosis is confirmed by biopsy.

Malignant melanoma is not sensitive to radiotherapy and the only hope of cure is by surgical removal. Survival after total rectal excision or local excision appears to be similar, with mean values ranging from 12 to 18 months.

Perianal Paget's Disease

Very rarely the perianal skin is affected by a scaling erythematous eczema histologically similar to that seen in Paget's disease of the nipple; this often indicates the presence of an underlying adenocarcinoma. The diagnosis is made on biopsy, which should include a sample of subcutaneous tissue. Treatment is by wide excision but rectal excision for an associated carcinoma may be necessary.

Bowen's Disease

Bowen's disease is a slow-growing intra-epidermal squamous cell carcinoma. It produces a chronic dermatosis not unlike Paget's disease and can also be mistaken for psoriasis, excoriation in pruritus ani or eczema.

The diagnosis is made by histological examination of a biopsy specimen and the treatment is excision of the affected skin. This may need to be extensive with skin grafting. The prognosis is good and if local recurrence develops, further local excision only is necessary.

Pilonidal Sinus

Pilonidal sinus is common and affects young adults, with males predominating in a ratio of about 3:1. It is rare in children and adolescents and in patients over the age of 40.

Definition

Pilonidal sinus is a chronic inflammatory lesion situated between the buttocks and consisting of one or more primary openings which communicate via the primary track with a subcutaneous cavity (Fig. 5.16). The primary track lies in

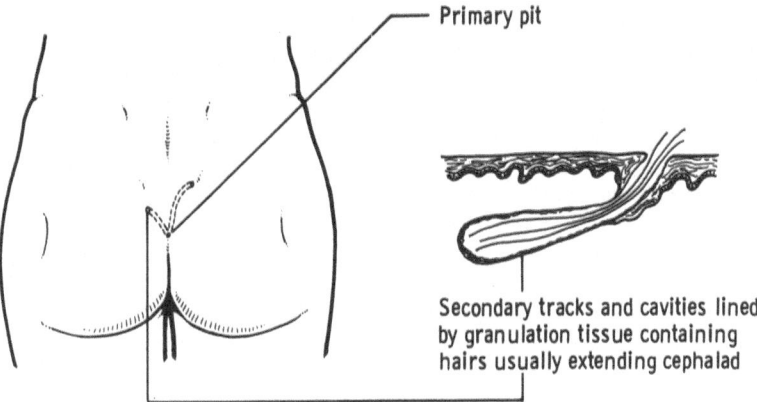

Fig. 5.16. Pilonidal sinus: primary pit and secondary tracks.

the natal cleft and is lined at its origin by cutaneous epithelium. This soon gives way to chronic inflammatory granulation tissue within the cavity, often containing foreign body giant cells. The cavity ramifies in various directions to open onto the surface via one or more secondary tracks. The primary tracks usually extend in a cephalad direction and the secondary openings are situated on either side of the midline, sometimes a considerable distance away.

Hairs are almost always found in the primary track. Some are detached and are lying loose but others may be rooted in hair follicles in the surrounding skin. Hair follicles are not present in the primary track.

Pathogenesis

For many years a congenital origin was accepted and numerous theories were proposed. All had one feature in common, namely the presence of an epithelial-lined abnormality in the natal cleft be it a pit or a subcutaneous cyst. Remnants of the medullary canal and dermoid inclusion cysts were postulated and it was also suggested that cutaneous pits could occur through retraction of the tail bud during embryological development. The persistent failure to find any epithelium within excised pilonidal sinuses examined histologically and the frequent observation that recurrence may occur after excision were the two most important pieces of evidence against the congenital theory.

It is now thought by many that an acquired cause is more likely. The presence of hairs in the primary track and the occurrence of pilonidal sinuses containing hairs elsewhere in the body—e.g. in the finger webs of barbers, at the umbilicus and in the axillae—suggests that the lesion starts by penetration of the skin by hairs. Most patients (but not all) are hirsute with considerable hair growth in the region of the sinus.

How penetration starts is not clear, however. In some cases it may be that the point of a hair still rooted in the surrounding area punctures the skin and is propelled deeper by the movement of the buttocks. However, more commonly the hairs found in the sinus are detached and are lying in the opposite direction, namely with their tips projecting from the opening. Some are too long to have originated from the immediate vicinity. It may be, therefore, that the penetration is made by loose hairs, for example from the head. Certainly this is consistent with the observation that a detached hair when gently rolled between a finger and the palm of the hand will tend to move in the direction of its root. This is due to the orientation of the scales on the hair, which project outwards from the shaft at an acute angle toward the tip. It may also be that there is some susceptibility of the skin to penetration by hairs.

Whatever the precise means of penetration, infection occurs leading to abscess formation in the subcutaneous tissue which may drain spontaneously via the primary site of entry or point elsewhere to form a secondary opening.

Diagnosis

The disease presents in two forms, namely as an acute abscess or as a chronic discharging sinus. The patient with a pilonidal abscess complains of a tender swelling in the natal cleft or buttock developing over a few days. Untreated it may settle spontaneously, but usually it bursts or is treated by surgical drainage. A chronic pilonidal sinus is then formed since healing of a discharged abscess is rare. The natural history of pilonidal sinus is characterised by relapses and remissions. The discharge may vary considerably and there is often recurrent abscess formation.

Pilonidal sinus may be confused with an anal fistula, hidradenitis suppurativa or a simple furuncle. It can be distinguished from an anorectal abscess first by its position and secondly by the absence of tenderness, swelling and induration in the immediate perianal region.

Treatment

A pilonidal abscess should be drained allowing the acute inflammation to settle. Cure is very unlikely and it is therefore necessary in most cases to deal with the resulting pilonidal sinus at a later date.

The treatment of a pilonidal sinus depends on the size of the lesion and the severity of symptoms. A small sinus which gives rise to only occasional discharge of a small amount of material can often be successfully managed by conservative means which include attention to hygiene, the removal of hairs from the track, and shaving the area or the application of epilatory creams.

In most cases, however, some form of operation is necessary. The various procedures described can be divided into two general types: those in which the whole lesion is widely excised and those in which the tracks are laid open and abscess cavities deroofed.

Wide Excision

For wide excision the anaesthetised patient is placed in the jack-knife or the left lateral position and the buttocks are strapped apart. An elliptical incision to include all primary and secondary openings is made and continued through the subcutaneous fat to the fascia over the sacrum and coccyx. The fat is separated from the fascia by sharp dissection and the specimen is removed. It may help to have previously injected dilute methylene blue into the sinus so that any track that has been opened by the dissection can be more easily identified.

The resulting wound may be left open to heal by secondary intention or closed by primary suture. With the former method healing takes a few weeks depending on the size of the wound but the patient can be ambulant for most of this time. A silicone foam stent (Silastic foam, Dow Corning) moulded to the shape of the cavity is a convenient dressing, new moulds being made as the wound gets smaller. During this time the wound edges should be kept shaved since hairs can grow into the wound and impede healing. The majority of cases heal satisfactorily by this method but recurrences occur in up to 10%. Simple primary suture may be suitable for small wounds but plastic techniques to close large defects without tension on the suture line have not become generally popular. It seems likely that the recurrence rate is higher after primary suture, with rates of around 20% or more having been reported.

Laying Open

In laying open a probe is inserted into the primary opening and an incision is made along its direction to open the track and main abscess cavity. Secondary tracks are laid open in a similar manner. After removal of hairs and curettage of granulation tissue, the wound edges are trimmed to obtain as flat a contour as possible to facilitate healing by secondary intention. With this method the resulting wound is smaller than with wide excision and the results are similar. In a more conservative variant of laying open, the primary and secondary openings are enlarged by circumcision and the cavity is cleaned by brushing or curettage, leaving the overlying skin intact. This operation can be carried out under local anaesthetic as an outpatient procedure. Provided the wound is correctly dressed and the skin shaved cure rates of 90% can be obtained.

Injection of the track with pure liquid phenol has been reported to produce satisfactory results in a similar proportion of patients.

Further Reading

FISSURE-IN-ANO

Bennett RC, Goligher JC (1962) Results of internal sphincterotomy for anal fissure. Br Med J II: 1500–1503

Crapp AR, Alexander-Williams J (1975) Fissure-in-ano and anal stenosis. I. Conservative manage-
    ment. Clin Gastroenterol 4: 619–628
Graham Stuart CW, Greenmore RK, Lloyd-Davies RW (1961) A review of 50 patients with fissure-
    in-ano. Surg Gynecol Obstet 113: 445–448
Hawley PR (1969) The treatment of chronic fissure-in-ano: A trial of methods. Br J Surg 56: 915–918
Hoffman DC, Goligher JC (1970) Lateral subcutaneous internal sphincterotomy in treatment of anal
    fissure. Br Med J III: 673–675
Keighley MRB, Greca F, Nevah E, Hares M, Alexander-Williams J (1981) Treatment of anal fissure
    by lateral and subcutaneous internal sphincterotomy should be under general anaesthesia. Br J
    Surg 68: 400–401
Lock MR, Thomson JPS (1977) Fissure-in-ano: The initial management and prognosis. Br J Surg 64:
    355–358
MacDonald P, Driscoll A, Nicholls RJ (1983) The anal dilator in the conservative management of
    acute anal fissures. Br J Surg 70: 25–26
Magee HR, Thompson HR (1966) Internal anal sphincterotomy as an outpatient operation. Gut 7:
    190–193
Marby M, Alexander-Williams J, Buchmann P, Arabi Y, Kappas A, Minervini S, Gatehouse D,
    Keighley MRB (1979) A randomised controlled trial to compare anal dilatation with lateral
    subcutaneous sphincterotomy for anal fissure. Dis Colon Rectum 22: 308–311
Millar DM (1971) Subcutaneous lateral internal sphincterotomy for anal fissure. Br J Surg 58:
    737–739
Notaras MJ (1971) The treatment of anal fissure by lateral subcutaneous internal sphincterotomy: A
    technique and results. Br J Surg 58: 96–100
Watts JM, Bennett RC, Goligher JC (1964) Stretching of anal sphincters in treatment of fissure-in-
    ano. Br Med J II: 342–343

HAEMORRHOIDS

Alexander-Williams J (1982) The nature of piles. Br Med J 285: 1064–1065
Ambrose NS, Hares MM, Alexander-Williams J, Keighley MRB (1983) Prospective randomised
    comparison of photocoagulation and rubber band ligation in treatment of haemorrhoids. Br Med
    J I: 1389–1391
Broader JH, Gunn IF, Williams JA (1974) Evaluation of a bulk forming evacuant in the management
    of haemorrhoids. Br J Surg 61: 142–144
Cheng FCY, Shum DWP, Ong GB (1981) The treatment of second degree haemorrhoids by
    injection, rubber band ligation, MDA and haemorrhoidectomy—a prospective clinical trial. Aust
    NZ J Surg 51: 458–462
Greca F, Hares MM, Nevah E, Williams JA, Keighley MRB (1981) A randomised trial to compare
    rubber band ligation with phenol injection of haemorrhoids. Br J Surg 68: 250–252
Groves AR, Evans JCW, Alexander-Williams J (1971) Management of internal haemorrhoids by
    rubber band ligation. Br J Surg 58: 923–924
Hancock B (1982) How do surgeons treat haemorrhoids? A study with special reference to Lord's
    procedure. Ann R Coll Surg Eng 64: 397–400
Hardy KJ, Wheatley IC, Heffernan EB (1975) Anal dilatation and haemorrhoidectomy: A prospec-
    tive study. Med J Aust 2: 88–91
Keighley MRB, Alexander-Williams J, Buchmann P et al. (1979) Prospective trials of minor surgical
    procedures and high fibre diet for haemorrhoids. Brit Med J II: 967–969
Leicester RJ, Nicholls RJ, Mann CV (1981) Infrared coagulation. A new treatment for haemorr-
    hoids. Dis Colon Rectum 24: 602–605
Leicester RJ (1983) Unpublished observations
Lord PH (1969) A day-case procedure for the cure of third-degree haemorrhoids. Br J Surg 56:
    747–749
Murie JA, Sim AJW, Mackenzie I (1981) The importance of pain, pruritus and soiling as symptoms
    of haemorrhoids and their response to haemorrhoidectomy or rubber band ligation. Br J Surg 68:
    247–249

Murie JA, Sim AJW, Mackenzie I (1982) Rubber band ligation versus haemorrhoidectomy for prolapsing haemorrhoids: A long term prospective clinical trial. Br J Surg 69: 536–538

O'Callaghan JD, Matheson TS, Hall R (1982) Inpatient treatment of prolapsing piles. Cryosurgery versus Milligan Morgan haemorrhoidectomy. Br J Surg: 157–159

Oh C (1981) One thousand cryohemorrhoidectomies: An overview. Dis Colon Rectum 24: 613–617

Sim AJW, Murie JA, Mackenzie I (1981) Comparison of rubber band ligation and sclerosant injection for 1st and 2nd degree haemorrhoids: A prospective clinical trial. Acta Chir Scand 147(8): 717–720

Templeton JL, Spence RAJ, Kennedy TL, Parks TG, Mackenzie G, Hanna WA (1983) Comparison of infrared coagulation for first and second degree haemorrhoids: A randomised prospective clinical trial. Br Med J I: 1387–1389

Thomson WHF (1975) The nature of haemorrhoids. Br J Surg 62: 542–552

Thomson WHF (1982) The real nature of 'perianal haematoma'. Lancet II: 467–468

Webster DJT, Gough DSC, Craven JL (1978) The use of bulk evacuant in patients with haemorrhoids. Br J Surg 65: 291–292

Wilson M, Schofield P (1976) Cryosurgical haemorrhoidectomy. Br J Surg 63: 497–498

ANORECTAL SEPSIS

Grace RH, Harper IA, Thompson RG (1982) Ano-rectal sepsis: Microbiology in relation to fistula-in-ano. Br J Surg 69: 401–403

Marks CG, Ritchie JK (1977) Anal fistulae at St Mark's Hospital. Br J Surg 64: 84–91

Oh C (1983) Management of high recurrent anal fistula. Surgery 93: 330–332

Parks AG (1961) Pathogenesis and treatment of fistula-in-ano. Br Med J I: 463–469

Parks AG, Thomson JPS (1983) Intersphincteric abscess. Br Med J II: 537–539

Parks AG, Gordon PH, Hardcastle JD (1976) A classification of fistula-in-ano. Br J Surg 63: 1–12

Stelzner F (1976) Die Anorectalen Fisteln, 2nd edn. Springer-Verlag, Berlin

ANAL CROHN'S DISEASE

Buchmann P, Keighley MRB, Allan RN, Thompson H, Alexander-Williams J (1980) Natural history of perianal Crohn's disease: A follow-up study. Am J Surg 140: 642–644

Hellers T, Bergstrand O, Ewerth S, Holstrom B (1980) Occurrence and outcome after primary treatment of anal fistulae in Crohn's disease. Gut 21: 525–527

Heuman R, Bolin T, Sjodahl R, Tagesson C (1981) The incidence and course of perianal complications and arthralgia after intestinal resection with restoration of continuity for Crohn's disease. Br J Surg 68: 528–530

Jeffrey PJ, Ritchie JK, Parks AG (1977) Treatment of haemorrhoids in patients with inflammatory bowel disease. Lancet I: 1084–1108

Marks CG, Ritchie JK, Lockhart-Mummery HE (1981) Anal fistulae in Crohn's disease. Br J Surg 68: 525–527

Sohn N, Forelitz BI, Weinstein MA (1980) Anorectal Crohn's disease: Definitive surgery for fistulas and recurrent abscesses. Am J Surg 139: 394–397

HIDRADENITIS SUPPURATIVA

Culp CE (1983) Chronic hidradenitis suppurativa of the anal canal. Dis Colon Rectum 26: 669–676

Goligher JC (1984) Surgery of the anus, rectum and colon, 5th edn. Baillière Tindall, London, pp 215–218

Morgan WP, Hughes LE (1979) The distribution, size and density of the apocrine glands in hidradenitis suppurativa. Br J Surg 66: 853–856

SEXUALLY TRANSMITTED DISEASES

Catterall RD (1975) Sexually transmitted diseases of the anus and rectum. Clin Gastroenterol 4: 659–669

Centers for Disease Control (1982) Sexually transmitted disease treatment guidelines. Morbidity and Mortality Weekly Report (Supplement) 31: 355–605

Crawford DH (1984) Lymphocyte and macrophage function. Br J Hosp Med 32: 112–115

Fauci AS, Macher AM, Londo DC et al. (1984) Acquired immunodeficiency syndrome: Epidemiology, clinical, immunologic and therapeutic considerations. Ann Intern Med 100: 92–106

Felman YM (1982) Sexually transmitted diseases in the male homosexual community. Cutis 30(6): 706, 710, 713–714

King A, Nicol C. Rodin P (1980) Venereal diseases, 4th edn. Baillière Tindall, London

Quinn TC, Corey L, Chaffee RG (1981), The etiology of anorectal infections in homosexual man. Am J Med 71: 345–406

Robbins RD, Sohn N, Weinstein MA (1983) Colorectal view of venereal disease. NY State J Med 83: 323–327

Thomson JPS, Grace R (1978) Perianal and anal condylomata acuminata: A new operative technique. J R Soc Med 71: 180–185

White FM (1983) Sexually transmitted diseases: Issues and priorities. Can Med Assoc J 128: 1178–1182

MALIGNANT ANAL TUMOURS

Cummings BJ (1982) The place of radiation therapy in the treatment of carcinoma of the anal canal. Cancer Treat Rev 9: 125–147

Nigro ND, Seydel HG, Cousidine B, Vaitkevicius VK, Leichman L, Kinzie J (1983) Combined preoperative radiation and chemotherapy for squamous cell carcinoma of the anal canal. Cancer 51: 1826–1829

Papillon J (1982) Rectal anal cancers: Conservative treatment by irradiation—an alternative to radical surgery. Springer-Verlag, Berlin

Papillon J, Mayer M, Montborbon JF, Gerard JP, Chassarol JL, Bailly C (1983) A new approach to the management of epidermoid carcinoma of the anal canal. Cancer 51: 1830–1837

Quan SHQ (1980) Uncommon malignant anal and rectal tumors. In: Stearns MW (ed) Neoplasms of the colon, rectum and anus. Wiley, New York

Rousseau J, Mathieu G, Fenton J (1979) Résultats et complications de la radiothérapie des epithéliomas du canal anal. Etude de 128 cas traités de 1956 à 1970. Gastroenterol Clin Biol (Paris) 3: 207–215

Stearns MW, Quan SHQ (1970) Epidermoid carcinoma of the anorectum. Surg Gynecol Obstet 131: 953–957

Wolfe HRI, Bussey HRJ (1968) Squamous cell carcinoma of the anus. Br J Surg 55: 295–301

PILONIDAL SINUS

Goligher JC (1984) Surgery of the anus, rectum and colon, 5th edn. Baillière Tindall, London, pp 221–236

Millar D (1981) Pilonidal sinus. In: Thomson JPS, Nicholls RJ, Williams CB (eds) Colorectal disease. Heinemann, London, pp 355–360

6 Pelvic Floor Disorders

Disorders of the pelvic floor include many cases of incontinence, complete rectal prolapse, mucosal prolapse and the solitary ulcer syndrome. Any of these can occur simultaneously and there are common aetiological factors linking them.

Descending Perineum Syndrome

A group of patients with abnormal descent of the perineum on bearing down has been defined, in whom a disorder of defaecation appears to be the initiating factor. Incomplete or difficult evacuation may cause the patient to strain leading to a prolonged reflex motor inhibition of the pelvic floor musculature and less rapid recovery of muscle tone. This results in abnormal descent of the perineum with associated bulging of the anterior rectal wall downwards towards the anal canal. It has been suggested that rectal mucosal prolapse then simulates a faecal bolus, giving the patient a persistent desire to defaecate. A vicious circle is set up in which descent and mucosal prolapse are aggravated by further straining (Fig. 6.1) which with time may lead to secondary neuromuscular damage to the pelvic floor. This complex of symptoms has been called the descending perineum syndrome.

The disorder is common and has been reported in 12% of a large consecutive series of patients attending a rectal clinic, of whom 80% complained of excessive straining and 70% spent more than 5 minutes in the lavatory each day.

Hypothesis

Abnormal perineal descent with associated neuropathic weakness of the pelvic

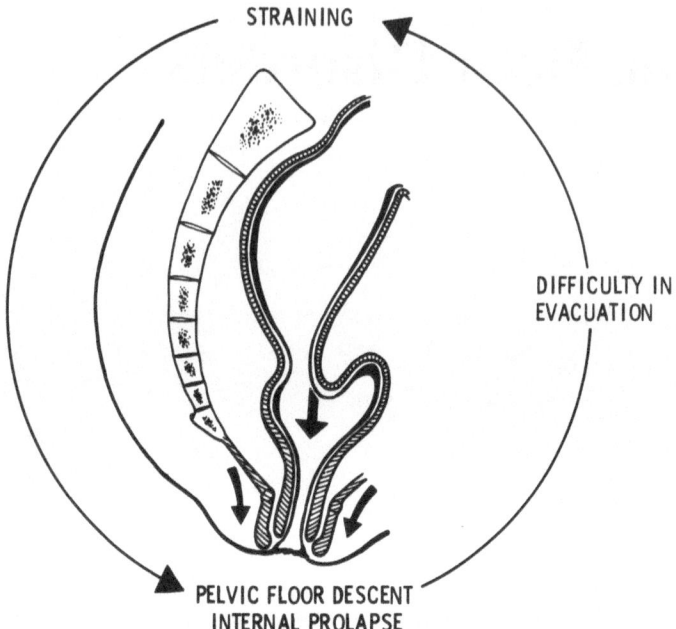

Fig. 6.1. The vicious circle: straining leading to pelvic floor descent and internal prolapse which causes further difficulty in defaecation.

floor musculature is common in rectal prolapse, anterior mucosal prolapse, neuropathic incontinence and in the solitary ulcer syndrome.

If abnormal perineal descent is one consequence of excessive straining, it is likely that internal rectal prolapse, mucosal or full thickness, is another. The histological appearances of rectal prolapse, mucosal prolapse and solitary ulcer are identical and they have many clinical features in common.

These associations can be integrated into a hypothesis (Table 6.1) in which straining initiated by difficulty in defaecation, leading to perineal descent and internal rectal prolapse, can then result in any of the pelvic floor disorders considered in this chapter. The reason for the initial difficulty in defaecation is unknown but the symptom in some cases is very likely to be one aspect of functional bowel disease. Symptoms of functional bowel disease are certainly common in patients with pelvic floor disorders.

Incontinence

The symptomatology, causes and assessment of incontinence have been dealt with in Chapter 4. In practice pelvic floor abnormalities leading to incontinence may cause a diffuse weakness of the pelvic musculature or a localised lesion. The former is due to neuropathic change while the latter is usually due to trauma causing disruption of the anal sphincter mechanism.

Table 6.1. Possible aetiological sequence in pelvic floor disorders

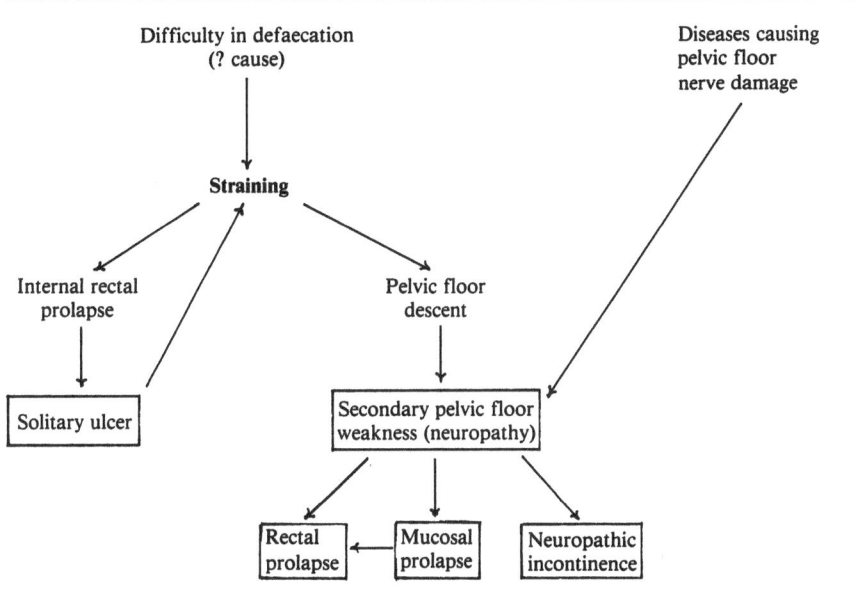

Pelvic Floor Neuropathy

In practice most patients with incontinence in whom diarrhoea is not responsible, present with a diffuse weakness of the anal sphincter mechanism and levator muscles. The anorectal angle widens (Fig. 6.2) and anal canal pressures are reduced. There is evidence in such cases to suggest damage to the nerve supply of these muscles. Histological studies have shown features of lower motor neurone denervation with abnormal fibre type grouping and muscle fibre hypertrophy. Single-fibre electromyography of the external anal sphincter has demonstrated an increase in the fibre density (i.e. the number of muscle fibres innervated by one axon) due to reinnervation of denervated muscle fibres by surviving axons, and estimation of the latency of the anal reflex has demonstrated an increase in patients with incontinence compared with controls. These physiological observations are consistent with denervation.

Most patients are female (sex ratio 9:1) and in some, incontinence occurs soon (weeks or months) after childbirth by vaginal delivery. There is now physiological evidence that some patients develop neuropathic changes in the pelvic floor musculature immediately after delivery. A history of difficulty in labour and the use of forceps is likely, and this taken with the association of the condition in

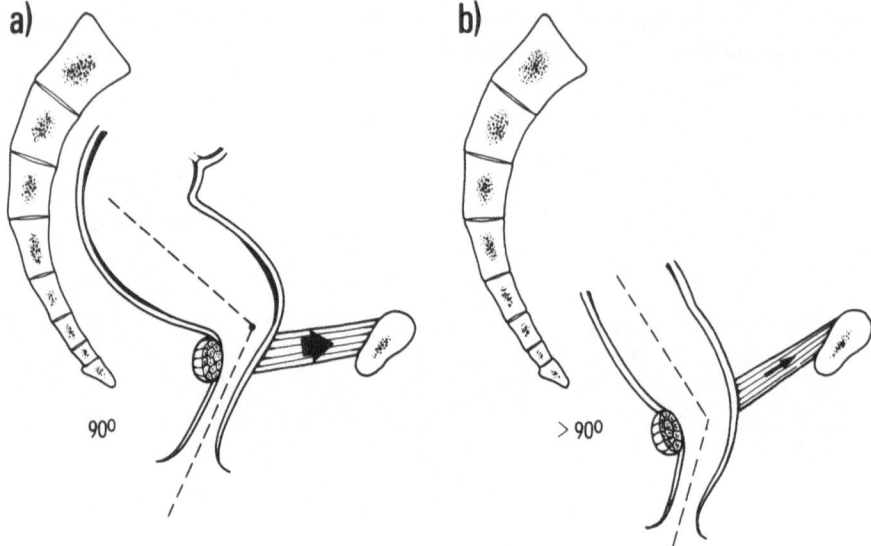

Fig. 6.2. Anorectal angle at rest: (a) normal; (b) with pelvic floor weakness.

other patients with defaecation difficulty and straining, has led to the suggestion that it may be due to traction or compression injury of the pudendal and sacral nerves innervating the pelvic floor.

Diagnosis

Symptoms and physical signs have already been considered (p.59).

Management

The indication for surgery depends on the severity of the incontinence. Some patients with loose stool may be adequately relieved by medication to thicken the consistency (codeine, loperamide), particularly if incontinence is infrequent. However, care should be taken to avoid causing constipation, which may lead to straining and even impaction. It may be helpful to prescribe evacuant suppositories to avoid this if the patient can retain them.

In other cases surgical repair is necessary. Post-anal repair of the pelvic floor aims to buttress the levators, restore the anorectal angle and elongate the anal canal, thereby giving the weakened musculature an improved mechanical advantage. Restoration of continence to normal or an acceptable level occurs in 65%–85% of cases and the clinical outcome can be related to improved anal manometric values measured postoperatively.

Pelvic Floor Trauma

The anal sphincter may be damaged by surgical operations (usually for fistula), obstetric trauma or non-iatrogenic trauma particularly road traffic accidents.

Surgical repair is indicated where incontinence is present and offers an excellent prospect of success, with restoration of continence in 85% or more of cases.

Solitary Ulcer Syndrome

In the nineteenth century non-malignant non-tuberculous ulcers in the rectum were reported from time to time. It was not until 1969, however, that the clinical features and pathology of the condition were described.

Solitary ulcer is said to be uncommon. On the basis of 51 cases presenting over a 10-year period in Northern Ireland, an incidence of 1 per 100 000 population per year was estimated. However, many of the symptoms which occur in the syndrome are fairly common, although rectal mucosal changes may be absent. The disease most often affects young adults, although the age range extends from childhood to old age; there is a tendency for it to be more common in females.

The term solitary ulcer is inaccurate since the lesions are often multiple and ulceration occurs in only half the cases.

Aetiology

There has been much speculation over causation. Some believe solitary ulcer to be due to self-abuse by instrumentation or anal intercourse but there is no evidence for this. Ischaemia has been proposed but the histological changes are not ischaemic in type.

It is more likely that the condition is due to internal rectal prolapse causing trauma to the rectal wall. The evidence in favour comes from the following observations. All patients give a history of straining at stool which in most cases can be identified as having preceded other symptoms such as bleeding and mucus. The straining seems to be in response to a feeling of incomplete evacuation of which all patients complain. Thus, there is a factor which would favour prolapse in every patient. Solitary ulcer is associated with abnormal perineal descent in about 50% of cases and often occurs with complete rectal prolapse, the reported coincidence ranging from 16% to 60%. The histological changes in solitary ulcer and complete rectal prolapse are furthermore identical. Sigmoidoscopic examination during straining frequently shows the lesion to descend towards the lumen of the instrument as evidence of internal rectal prolapse. This is particularly pronounced if the biopsy window is removed, opening the rectal lumen to atmospheric pressure. A similar observation can be made on proctoscopy. In cases without overt rectal prolapse, an abdominal mobilisation of the rectum anteriorly with fixation using a foreign implant markedly reduces the feeling of tenesmus. Where rectal prolapse is present, the solitary ulcer seems to be cured by a successful rectopexy.

About 50% of patients with solitary ulcer show contraction (rather than relaxation) of the puborectalis when making straining efforts to defaecate. There is also a high incidence of pelvic floor neuropathic changes judged by fibre density estimations and delayed pudendal nerve conduction times.

Thus it may well be that a solitary ulcer starts through difficulty in evacuation leading to habitual straining which causes internal rectal prolapse and secondary neuropathic damage to the pelvic floor. Damage to the rectum occurs as the prolapse is pushed down against a paradoxically contracting pelvic floor and the presence of the prolapse itself exacerbates the feeling of incomplete evacuation leading to an increase in straining efforts to defaecate.

Diagnosis

Symptoms

Almost all patients complain of difficulty in defaecation associated with a feeling of incomplete evacuation and a persistent desire to void. Although the patient's bowels may be open once or twice a day it is common to find this to be the result of several fruitless visits to the lavatory of 10–20 minutes each; in a few patients half an hour or more may be spent there on each occasion. Simply asking the patient the frequency of defaecation may miss this typical and important symptom. Many assist defaecation by digitation. Almost all complain of bleeding and the passage of mucus and some of incontinence and pain. The pain is difficult to define, but it seems to be located deep in the perineum. Straining worsens the symptoms which in turn exacerbate the desire to defaecate leading to further straining. A vicious circle is thus created.

Some patients also complain of abdominal symptoms including pain and distension typical of irritable bowel syndrome. Some are neurotic, but whether this is a cause or effect of the symptoms is not clear. Indeed, the symptoms may be so severe as to dominate the patient's life.

Signs

Abnormal descent of the perineum on straining is present in about 50% of cases. The oedematous ulcerated mucosa may be felt on digital examination as a hard, often tender, localised lesion, occasionally indistinguishable from a carcinoma. Four typical signs are usually found on sigmoidoscopy, namely mucus and blood in the lumen, and redness and oedema of an area of mucosa. The lesion is often seen on the fold of a valve of Houston and ulceration is evident in about 50% of cases. In about 20% the mucosa has a marked polypoid appearance and a stricture may be present. The majority (70%) of solitary ulcers lie anteriorly at

7-10 cm from the anal verge; only 20% are posterior and 10% circumferential. A full thickness rectal prolapse may also be present.

Investigation

A biopsy is essential to exclude carcinoma. Histological abnormalities include increased numbers of fibroblasts in the lamina propria, dense fibrosis in the submucosa, hypertrophy of the muscularis mucosae, and epithelial regeneration at the edge of the ulcer with mucin depletion. These changes are the same as those seen in complete and mucosal rectal prolapse.

Tests of anorectal physiology do not contribute to the diagnosis but may be helpful in assessing the sphincter mechanism in cases of incontinence. They have also been valuable in studying the nature of the disease.

Management

Abdominal rectopexy is indicated in patients with simultaneous complete rectal prolapse. Healing rates after this procedure of over 80% have been reported. Straining and constipation afterwards should be avoided if possible.

In cases without prolapse, however, the management is less straightforward. Conservative treatment consists of trying to prevent straining by explanation, exhortation and prescribing suppositories (e.g. glycerine or bisacodyl) to facilitate a strain-free evacuation. This regime rarely works, largely because patients find it very difficult in practice to stop straining and answering the frequent call to stool. Surgical excision of the ulcerated area is followed by recurrence but the ulcer has been observed to heal following a colostomy in the few cases treated, only to recur, however, after subsequent closure. Initial experience with a modified rectopexy aimed at reducing mobility of the anterior rectal wall has been encouraging. The feeling of incomplete evacuation has been abolished in all cases treated, with improvement of other symptoms in 80%.

Rectal Prolapse

Rectal prolapse may be complete, when the entire thickness of the rectal wall is involved, or partial, when only the mucosa prolapses.

Complete Rectal Prolapse

Rectal prolapse may occur in infancy or young adult life, but is far more common in old age. The sex ratio of patients is roughly equal up to 65 years, after which it is ten times commoner in females.

Aetiology

Rectal prolapse is associated with two abnormalities, namely a weak pelvic floor and a mobile rectum.

WEAK PELVIC FLOOR. The condition can be produced in exerimental animals by division of the nerves to the pelvic floor muscles and sometimes occurs in patients with cauda equina lesions or neurological diseases such as disseminated sclerosis. Anorectal physiological studies show evidence of a pelvic floor neuropathy in 70% of patients and faecal incontinence is common. The increasing frequency of rectal prolapse with age is in parallel with the progressive neuropathy of the pelvic floor, which accelerates after 65 years in the normal population. Although injury during childbirth may cause pelvic floor weakness, childbirth per se is probably not associated with most cases of prolapse since 50% of women presenting with prolapse in old age are nulliparous.

MOBILE RECTUM. Evidence of increased rectal mobility comes from observations made during laparotomy. The rectovaginal or rectovesical pouch is deep, with extensive peritoneal covering of the lateral aspect of the rectum and the presence of a rectal mesentery in some cases. The sigmoid colon and rectosigmoid are redundant. Thus there is less extraperitoneal rectum than normal.

The combination of a mobile rectum and a weak pelvic floor leads to prolapse either by a sliding mechanism or through intussusception, and both probably occur in practice.

Many patients admit to excessive straining at stool. While this could well tip the balance in favour of prolapse in a patient with an already compromised pelvic floor, straining weakens the musculature in time and is likely to be an important factor in causation. Some patients give a long history of constipation, others of self-neglect with episodes of impaction. Some, particularly in the younger age group, are mentally deficient or have personality disorders. They may be in institutions where for both physical and mental reasons straining is perhaps more prevalent and encouraged by the constipation produced by many antidepressants. Prolapse is common among members of a religious sect in Central Europe in which straining is performed as part of a ritual observance. Rectal prolapse is associated with the solitary ulcer syndrome, where straining is a common feature.

Pathology

Prolapse causes trauma of the mucosa leading to ulceration and haemorrhage with increased mucus production.

Diagnosis

SYMPTOMS. In infants the mother will see the prolapse, which bleeds and produces excessive mucus. The child is usually otherwise fit, eating well and gaining weight.

Adults are often reticent about their disease, particularly if they are incontinent as well, and may suffer in secrecy before seeking help. The history may therefore be long-standing, occasionally years.

The prolapse may only descend during defaecation and reduce spontaneously afterwards or it may require replacement by the patient. In more severe cases it occurs on standing or walking and sometimes it is present all the time. The rectal mucosa secretes mucus and bleeds and about 50% of patients complain of faecal incontinence. Sometimes this is the main presenting symptom and the patient may not have been aware of any prolapse.

SIGNS. The mental state of the patient should be noted and an assessment of the general physical condition made. Signs of neurological disease should be looked for, particularly in the lower limbs and around the anus.

The diagnosis is made on inspection by demonstrating the prolapse. Often it is necessary to ask the patient to bear down to do so. Sometimes it can be produced only when the patient strains while standing. Weakness of the pelvic floor is manifested by abnormal perineal descent on straining, poor voluntary contraction of the levators, puborectalis and external sphincter and poor anorectal angle. Resting anal canal tone is usually low, and a patulous anus can be demonstrated in almost all patients by gently parting the anal verge.

Sigmoidoscopy must be carried out in all patients since occasionally a carcinoma is also present. It is often unsatisfactory, however, since the sphincter may be too weak to retain insufflated air.

Haemorrhoids, mucosal prolapse and polyps in the lower rectum (especially if large and sessile) may simulate rectal prolapse and the reddening on sigmoidoscopy may suggest proctitis. Any suspicious lesion should be biopsied. Intussusception in infants can be distinguished from prolapse on digital examination, whereby the finger enters the rectum lateral to the intussuscipiens.

Investigation

Investigation of the colon is indicated where there is clinical suspicion of proximal disease. Assessment of incontinence by anorectal physiological tests, if available, gives an objective record of sphincter function.

Management

In infancy the treatment should be conservative, avoiding straining by preventing constipation and encouraging the mother to pot the child for short periods when bowel training is started. The mother should replace the prolapse when it occurs. Usually this treatment is successful but injection of the prolapse with sclerosant may help in a few difficult cases.

In adults the treatment is surgical. Abdominal rectopexy, in which the rectum is mobilised posteriorly and laterally, gives 5-year cure rates of 90%–95%. Various techniques with or without the use of foreign implants have been described. The operation is well tolerated by old people. Most cases of recurrent prolapse can be treated by a second rectopexy. Perineal operations, of which there are many types, give relatively less long-lasting relief with recurrence rates of 30% or more. Thiersch wire or silastic loop insertion operations lead to a high incidence of faecal impaction and infection and often do not help incontinence or control the prolapse.

About 50% of patients who have both incontinence and prolapse regain continence after an abdominal rectopexy. In those who fail to do so, a perineal pelvic floor repair should be attempted provided the prolapse has been dealt with successfully.

Mucosal Prolapse

Redundant mucosa of the lower rectum may be forced into the anal canal on straining. It can present as an overt prolapse seen emerging from the anus or it may be occult and detectable only by proctoscopy.

As would be expected, mucosal prolapse is often associated with prolapsing haemorrhoids and some cases probably represent a precursor of complete rectal prolapse. Thus there may be evidence of pelvic floor weakness especially perineal descent.

Diagnosis

SYMPTOMS. The symptoms are identical to those produced by haemorrhoids, and include mucous leakage, bleeding, prolapse, pruritis ani and discomfort. Discomfort may predominate and is often described as a sensation of heaviness or even of a lump deep in the perineum. Often there is a feeling of incomplete evacuation with frequent fruitless visits to the lavatory, as occurs in the solitary ulcer syndrome.

SIGNS. Some mucosal descent on straining, especially of the anterior rectal wall, is probably normal on proctoscopy since it can be demonstrated in the majority of patients. The diagnosis of occult mucosal prolapse may therefore be made more often than is justified by the symptoms since assessment of the degree of prolapse is subjective. Perineal descent and weakness of the anal sphincter are present in some cases. The prolapsing mucosa is often reddened and sometimes can be seen to be producing mucus. There may also be ulceration and bleeding. Haemorrhoids are usually present.

The differential diagnosis is the same as for complete rectal prolapse.

Investigation

No special investigations are required. Biopsy is necessary only when the diagnosis is in doubt. Histological changes are the same as those in rectal prolapse and solitary ulcer.

Management

Management includes measures to induce defaecation without straining and local treatment of the prolapse. The nature of the condition should be explained to the patient and the need to avoid straining emphasised. The aim should be to try and establish a regular pattern of defaecation once or twice a day without intervening visits to the lavatory. In some patients this can be achieved by means of evacuant suppositories taken at a specific time during the day. The patient is told that having emptied the rectum there should be no need to defaecate for 12 or 24 hours whatever sensation is felt in the perineum. If the call to stool is resisted and the time spent in the lavatory is kept to a minimum, straining may be avoided with some hope of improvement. If the stool is hard, bulk laxatives or bran should be prescribed. Too much can, however, increase stool volume and frequency may be made worse. Local treatment of the prolapse includes injection sclerotherapy or rubber band ligation. There is no information available on how often this regime is successful. Without doubt some patients are helped but recurrence of symptoms after a few weeks or months is very common. In some patients with severe persistent symptoms operative removal of the prolapse has been undertaken, but again little is known about the results.

Further Reading

Bartolo DC, Read NW, Jarratt JA, Read MG, Donnelly TC, Johnson AG (1983) Differences in anal sphincter function and clinical presentation in patients with pelvic floor descent. Gastroenterology 85: 68–75

Beersiek F, Parks AG, Swash M (1979) Pathogenesis of ano-rectal incontinence: A histometric study of the anal sphincter musculature. J Neurol Sci 42: 111–127

Bennett RC, Duthie HL (1964) The functional importance of the internal anal sphincter. Br J Surg 51: 355–357

Broden B, Snellman B (1968) Procidentia of the rectum studied with cine radiography: A contribution to the discussion of causative mechanisms. Dis Colon Rectum 11: 330–347

Browning GGP, Parks AG (1983) Postanal repair for neuropathic faecal incontinence. Correlation of clinical results and anal canal pressures. Br J Surg 20: 101–104

Duthie HL (1982) Defaecation and the anal sphincters. Clin Gastroenterol 11: 621–631

Goldberg SM, Gordon PH, Nivatvongs S (1980) Essentials of anorectal surgery. Lippincott, Philadelphia

Henry MM, Parks AG, Swash M (1982) The pelvic floor musculature in the descending perineum syndrome. Br J Surg 53: 760–765

Keighley MRB, Fielding JWL (1983) Management of faecal incontinence and results of surgical treatment. Br J Surg 70: 463–468

Keighley MRB, Fielding JL, Alexander-Williams J (1983) Results of abdominal rectopexy using polypropylene (Marlex) mesh in 100 consecutive patients. Br J Surg 70: 229–232

Kerremans R (1969) Morphological and physiological aspects of anal continence and defaecation. Arscia Vitgaven, Brussels

Madigan MR, Morson BC (1969) Solitary ulcer of the rectum. Gut 10: 871–881

Martin CJ, Parks TG, Biggart JD (1981) Solitary rectal ulcer syndrome in Northern Ireland 1971–80. Br J Surg 68: 744–747

Neill ME, Parks AG, Swash M (1981) Physiological studies of the anal sphincter musculature in faecal incontinence and rectal prolapse. Br J Surg 68: 531–536

Parks AG (1975) Anorectal incontinence. Proc Soc Med 68: 681–690
Parks AG, McPartlin JF (1977) Surgical repair of anal sphincters following injury. In: Todd IP (ed)
    Colon, rectum and anus (3rd edn Operative surgery). Butterworth, London, pp 245–248
Parks AG, Porter NH, Hardcastle JD (1966) The syndrome of the descending perineum. Proc Soc
    Med 59: 477–482
Rutter KPR, Riddell RH (1975) The solitary ulcer syndrome of the rectum. Clin Gastroenterol 4:
    505–530
Schweiger M, Alexander-Williams J (1977) Solitary ulcer syndrome of the rectum: Its association
    with occult rectal prolapse. Lancet I: 170
Snooks SJ, Setchell ME, Swash M, Henry MM (1984) Injury to innervation of pelvic floor sphincter
    musculature in childbirth. Lancet II: 546–550
White CM, Findlay JM, Price JJ (1980) The occult rectal prolapse syndrome. Br J Surg 67: 528–530

7 Polyps

A polyp is a localised elevated lesion arising from an epithelial surface, and may be pedunculated or sessile. Polyps of the large bowel and rectum are common and are found in about 10% of patients presenting to a rectal clinic. They can occur as solitary lesions, synchronously in small numbers or as part of a polyposis syndrome. Before the advent of the double contrast barium enema examination, many polyps were probably missed. The introduction of the colonoscope has further increased the diagnostic yield and has profoundly influenced the treatment and management of such patients.

The most useful classification is pathological (Table 7.1), as the histological type determines management. The important distinction is between neoplastic and non-neoplastic polyps. Neoplastic polyps can be benign or malignant. A benign polyp is referred to as an adenoma and a malignant polyp as an adenocarcinoma. The adenoma is important as it is potentially malignant.

Non-neoplastic Polyps

Metaplastic polyps are common, occurring in 5%–10% of patients examined by sigmoidoscopy. They develop as a deformity of the normal bowel epithelium in which there is cystic dilation and elongation of the crypts. The cells themselves are indistinguishable from normal large bowel epithelial cells. Metaplastic polyps are thought to have no malignant potential, their importance being that they may be confused with adenomas.

Inflammatory polyps may be found in colitis and any condition where ulceration has occurred. They are formed by oedematous processes of mucosa between areas of ulceration.

Table 7.1. Classification of polyps of the large bowel and rectum (WHO)

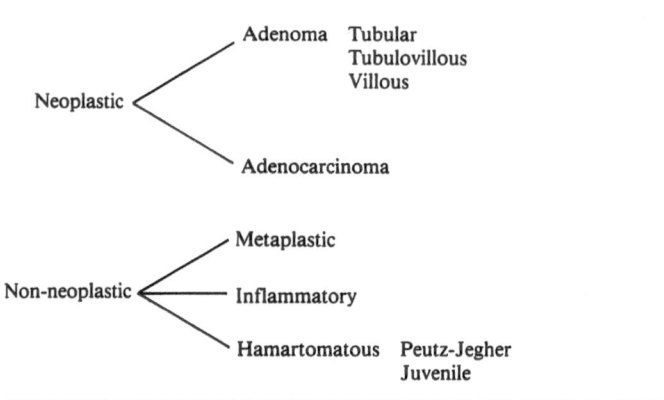

Hamartomatous polyps are rare and occur in two forms, namely as juvenile polyps and in the Peutz-Jegher syndrome. Although different histologically they share the common features of hamartomas, which include the presence of morphologically normal epithelial cells arranged within an excessive connective tissue stroma. Juvenile polyps occur in children and young adults: they may be sporadic when few in number or genetic when they are multiple. Peutz-Jegher polyps can also occur genetically as a polyposis syndrome and are most numerous in the small bowel.

Neoplastic Polyps

Adenoma

An adenoma begins in one area of a crypt as a proliferation of epithelial cells which show increased staining of nuclei, pleomorphism and mitoses, features referred to as dysplasia. In normal epithelium the nuclei lie consistently at the base of the cell adjacent to the basement membrane. In an adenoma this regular arrangement is lost and the nuclei are found at variable points between the base and apex of the cells (loss of stratification of the nuclei).

There are two basic types of adenoma: tubular and villous (Fig. 7.1). A tubular adenoma consists of compactly arranged tubules (resulting from excessive branching of the normal crypt glands) surrounded by stroma. In a villous adenoma epithelial proliferation occurs outwards into the lumen as frond-like neoplastic processes with the stroma lying as a core within the epithelial elements. In a tubulovillous adenoma both morphological patterns occur.

Tubular and villous adenomas tend to differ in their macroscopic appearances. The former are usually pedunculated, the latter sessile. Villous adenomas are on the whole more extensive and involve a greater area of mucosa than tubular adenomas. Malignant change is more likely to occur in villous adenomas.

Adenomas are frequently multiple, the term synchronous being used to describe other coexisting lesions. However, it is uncommon for there to be more than five or so synchronous adenomas in any given individual except in the rare

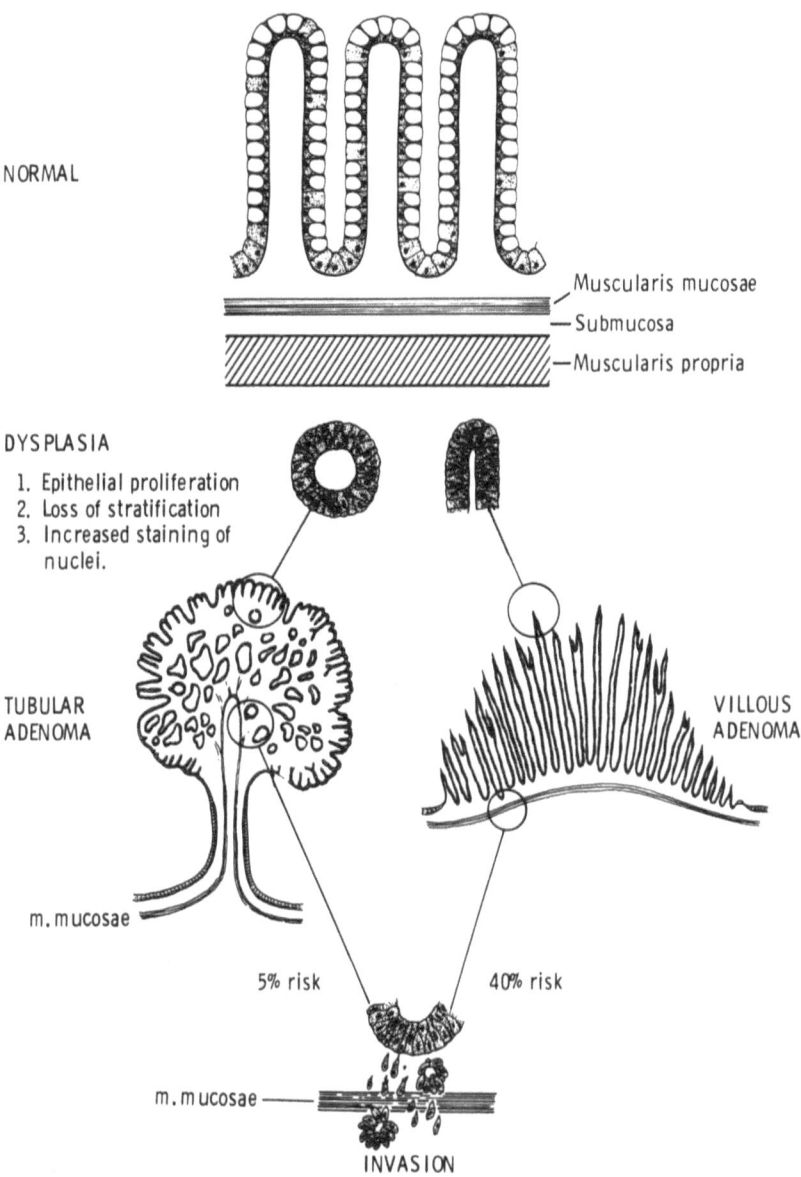

Fig. 7.1. The architecture of tubular and villous adenomas: morphology of invasion.

condition of familial adenomatosis where hundreds or even thousands may be present. When one adenoma has formed, there is a tendency for further (metachronous) adenomas to develop in the future.

Carcinomatous Change

There is much evidence to suggest that most carcinomas develop within a pre-existing adenoma (Table 7.2). However, this sequence may not apply to all carcinomas and certainly those that develop in ulcerative colitis usually do not appear to be preceded by an adenoma stage.

Table 7.2. Evidence for adenoma–carcinoma sequence

Clinical evidence	Histopathological evidence
Synchronous adenomas occur in about 30% of patients with large bowel cancer	Cellular appearances of adenoma and well-differentiated carcinoma are identical
Distribution of adenomas and carcinomas in bowel is similar	Malignant change is frequently seen in adenomas and is related to size of adenoma
Incidence of metachronous carcinoma is doubled if an adenoma was present in original resection specimen	Adenomatous tissue is commonly seen around carcinoma, more frequently with Dukes A (30%) than with Dukes C lesions (5%)
There is an association between adenoma and carcinoma in familial adenomatous polyposis	
Peak age incidence of adenoma precedes that of carcinoma by about 5 years	
Regular identification and removal of adenomas may reduce incidence of carcinoma	

Although an adenoma contains dysplastic cells it only becomes a carcinoma when cells invade through the muscularis mucosae into the submucosa. Penetration of the muscularis mucosae is the only criterion used by the pathologist to diagnose carcinoma and the term carcinoma-in-situ should not be used; the neoplasm is either an adenoma or a carcinoma (Fig. 7.1).

Having invaded the submucosa, the carcinoma spreads by direct extension, penetrating the bowel wall to involve extramural fat and surrounding organs. During this process it invades blood vessels and lymphatics and by permeation and embolisation causes blood-borne and lymphatic metastases. Invasion through to the peritoneal serosa may be followed by transcoelomic spread.

The histological appearances vary from well differentiated, where tubule formation is well developed and cellular morphology resembles the normal, to poorly differentiated, where tubular architecture is absent and the cells are grossly aberrant. Most carcinomas show a degree of differentiation between these extremes.

Clinical Features

Symptoms

In patients with an adenoma the presence of symptoms is related to the size of the lesion. Most adenomas less than 10 mm in diameter are asymptomatic and are found incidentally on endoscopy or barium enema examination. With large polyps the commonest symptom is bleeding, which usually occurs intermittently and in small amounts; a brisk bleed is very unlikely to be due to an adenoma. As with carcinoma, it is now well established, from screening studies using faecal occult blood testing, that bleeding is often unnoticed by the patient. Bleeding from a colonic adenoma is typically dark red and mixed with stool. An adenoma in the rectum may, however, lead to the passage of bright unmixed blood indistinguishable in type from that produced by anal disorders such as haemorrhoids.

Patients with large bowel adenomas may notice mucus in the stool. Its presence is of little value in differential diagnosis since it may also be seen with carcinoma and other diseases such as colitis, diverticular disease, rectal prolapse and haemorrhoids. However, villous adenomas of the rectum and distal sigmoid colon may produce large amounts of mucus, which is usually of a watery consistency and can occasionally amount to several hundred millilitres per day. Fluid and potassium depletion is classically described in this condition but is in fact exceedingly rare.

Diarrhoea may occur in some patients with adenoma. This is probably the result of the admixture of mucus and faeces resulting in a fluid stool.

Juvenile polyps produce mucus with a yellowish hue. They are pedunculated with a stalk which is weak and slender since it is devoid of muscularis mucosae. There is a tendency therefore for torsion to occur, leading to sloughing of the polyp (autoamputation). The shed polyp may be seen within the stool by the patient or patient's mother.

In patients with Peutz-Jegher polyps the most common symptom is abdominal pain resulting from small bowel intussusception as the polyp is propelled by peristalsis. Such polyps do not usually bleed.

Inflammatory polyps produce no special symptoms, but they are an indication of severe damage to the mucosa from inflammatory bowel disease. Metaplastic polyps are asymptomatic.

Signs

Benign polyps vary in size from a few millimetres to several centimetres. Those less than 5 mm in diameter are generally hemispherical or tag-like and do not usually have a stalk, since they have not yet grown sufficiently to form one. Such polyps are usually metaplastic or small adenomas.

A pedunculated polyp has a head and a stalk. The head of an adenoma is usually pinkish-red, contrasting with the more yellow colour of the normal mucosa. The stalk varies in length from a few millimetres to some centimetres; if long, the polyp will be very mobile within the lumen. The head is composed of dysplastic tissue and the stalk of attenuated normal mucosa and muscularis mucosae. Endoscopic evidence of a thickened or rigid stalk suggests that malignant invasion may have occurred. Ulceration of the head is not evident in a benign adenoma although blood in the lumen may be present.

A sessile polyp is less easily definable. It appears as a projection of exuberant tissue into the lumen but lacks a pedicle. Most sessile polyps are villous adenomas, some of which contain malignant foci. Macroscopic ulceration is usually absent unless frank carcinoma is present. The lesion may, however, extend over large areas and is more common in the rectum than in other parts of the bowel. Mucus is usually present in the lumen.

Digital palpation per rectum is clearly only appropriate to lesions within range of the examining finger, i.e. up to about 12 cm from the anal verge. Small polyps of less than 5 mm are usually impalpable but larger pedunculated polyps may be felt as mobile swellings. They are usually soft owing to a lack of fibrous tissue within them, and may easily be missed. Like pedunculated adenomas, sessile adenomas feel soft, but if an area of hardness is present invasion into the submucosa is likely to have occurred. The hardness is due to the desmoplastic reaction around the malignant focus. Digital examination is essential in assessing rectal polyps since it is the best means of detecting malignant change.

Identification of Malignant Change in Adenomas

While in some cases it is only possible to identify malignant change on microscopic examination of the excised adenoma, a number of features may suggest the possibility before removal (Table 7.3):

Size: There is a high chance of malignant foci being present in adenomas over 25 mm in diameter.

Morphology: Villous adenomas are more likely to have malignant foci than tubular adenomas.

Ulceration: The presence of ulceration favours malignancy.

Table 7.3. Risk (%) of malignant change being found in adenomas removed by colonoscopy

Diameter of adenoma (mm)	Type of adenoma		
	Tubular	Tubulovillous	Villous
< 10	0–1	0–1	0–1 (10)[a]
10–25	3	4	5 (10)
> 25	10	11	38 (53)

[a] Figures in brackets show the risk of malignant change in *surgically* removed rectal villous tumours.

Hardness: Hardness detected on palpation usually indicates malignancy unless other factors, e.g. scarring due to previous diathermy fulguration, can explain it.

Indrawing of the base: Distortion of the contour of the bowel wall seen on the barium enema examination suggests invasion.

Diagnosis and Management

The histological type is the most important factor influencing management. Since there may be more than one polyp, or an associated cancer in patients with an adenoma, a polyp should not be removed until the entire colon and rectum have been examined. If no cancer is present all polyps can then be removed, combining treatment with diagnosis.

The clinical steps in management therefore include identification of a polyp, identification of synchronous polyps, removal for histological diagnosis, taking a family history and follow-up.

Identification

A polyp is usually seen either on the initial sigmoidoscopy or on a barium enema examination. Up to a few years ago rigid sigmoidoscopy was the only means of inspecting the large bowel mucosa, but with the introduction of flexible sigmoidoscopy for outpatient use more polyps are being identified on the first consultation.

Small non-pedunculated polyps show on barium enema examination as a ring shadow which must be distinguished from faecal and air bubble shadows. When seen side on, the head and stalk of a pedunculated polyp are usually clearly apparent as separate shadows in continuity. In an en face view, pedunculated polyps may give rise to two concentric shadows, the outer representing the head, the inner the stalk. A sessile polyp produces a filling defect over an area corresponding to its base. In the absence of malignant change the contour of the normal bowel shadow on each side of the polyp is in linear continuity. Where malignant change has occurred, this line becomes irregular due to drawing in of the base by fibrosis resulting from the desmoplastic reaction.

Synchronous Polyps

Having identified a polyp the next stage is to determine the number present. If one has not already been carried out, the most effective way of doing so is by double contrast barium enema examination. This technique provides excellent mucosal definition and about 90% of polyps less than 5 mm in diameter can be identified. Lesions may however be missed from time to time, particularly if the bowel is poorly prepared or when the lesions are located in the sigmoid colon where overlapping of bowel and distortion due to diverticular disease may impair mucosal definition.

Colonoscopy should be reserved for those patients in whom contrast radiology is unsatisfactory or is negative but where clinical features suggest that further lesions exist.

Occasionally hundreds of polyps may be demonstrated, indicating a polyposis syndrome (see below). A few other patients may be found to have a carcinoma.

Removal

The method of removal depends on the site and the morphology of the polyp (i.e. whether pedunculated or sessile).

Pedunculated polyps can be removed by snare excision, either via the rigid sigmoidoscope if they are in the rectum or by colonoscopic snare polypectomy if they are more proximal. Colonoscopy has the advantage that all synchronous lesions can be excised simultaneously. Small polyps of a few millimetres in diameter can be entirely removed during rigid sigmoidoscopy using large cusp forceps or on colonoscopy by the hot biopsy technique in which the polyp is partially biopsied (obtaining tissue for histology) and the remnant destroyed simultaneously by diathermy applied via the biopsy forceps.

Sessile polyps in the lower and mid rectum should be carefully palpated for areas of hardness indicating malignant change. If none is present submucosal excision via an anal retractor should be carried out. Large sessile polyps covering many square centimetres can be removed by this technique and every effort should be made to preserve the specimen intact, taking the lesion with a surrounding margin of normal mucosa.

Sessile polyps in the upper rectum and colon can be removed by snare polypectomy if they are less than 25 mm in diameter, by applying traction on the lesion to create a false pedicle. This technique is dangerous for larger polyps, risking perforation or incomplete removal, and these require laparotomy and resection of bowel.

Histological Diagnosis

The pathologist has two tasks: first to make a histological diagnosis and secondly to determine in the case of adenomas whether malignant invasion has taken place. As a general principle, therefore, a polyp should be removed by complete excision biopsy so that surrounding normal tissue containing muscularis mucosae is present. With a pedunculated polyp it is important to remove some of the stalk along with the head. With a sessile polyp the specimen should be removed intact and have a surrounding margin of normal mucosa. In this circumstance it is most helpful to the pathologist if the specimen is fixed to resemble its configuration in vivo. The surgeon can assist by pinning the specimen out on to a cork board directly after removal to minimise contraction and distortion before fixation. If pots of formalin are kept in the operating theatre they should be big enough to accommodate these specimens.

All polyps must be numbered and sent to the pathologist in labelled pots and their corresponding sites recorded on a diagram in the hospital notes. The location of any that have undergone malignant change will thus be known.

Follow-up

The need for further action depends on the histological type of the polyp. A patient with a metaplastic polyp need not be followed, but those with hamarto-matas and adenomas should be. Patients with adenomas are at increased risk of developing metachronous adenomas and carcinoma. This is cumulative over the years and probably amounts respectively to about 40% and 10% over a 20-year period. The risk appears to be greater if synchronous adenomas were originally present and if the patient was over 60 years at initial diagnosis. There is a suggestion that a family history of large bowel cancer also increases the risk.

The optimal frequency of follow-up and method of examination have not been established and it is not yet known whether an adenoma follow-up system is effective in cancer prevention. At the present time certain centres recommend a full examination of the large bowel, preferably by colonoscopy, at 1–3 years after identifying an adenoma, the exact interval depending on risk factors. There is, however, a logistic problem since adenomas are common and regular surveillance of the large bowel of all such patients may well stretch medical services while giving a possibly useful yield in only a few cases.

Family History

A family history must be taken from patients with hamartomatous polyps and adenomas since there is always the possibility of a polyposis syndrome, all of which have a dominant mode of inheritance. It may be, however, that there is an increased familial incidence of bowel neoplasia in patients with so-called sporadic adenomas.

Malignant Colorectal Polyps

The risks of an invasive cancer developing in an adenoma have already been discussed. The majority of malignant polyps can be successfully treated by polypectomy alone (either by snare or local excision) provided that the specimen is carefully examined and that certain histopathological criteria are strictly applied.

If the lesion has been completely excised and is not found to be poorly differentiated, no further action is needed except careful follow-up by colono-scopy. Malignant polyps uncommonly contain poorly differentiated carcinoma but the risk of lymph node metastasis is significant in such cases. If, therefore, the lesion is poorly differentiated or is incompletely excised surgical resection is necessary.

Polyposis Syndromes

Peutz-Jegher Polyposis

The diagnosis of Peutz-Jegher polyposis is made by the demonstration of small bowel polyps after a small bowel barium meal and the identification of typical circumoral and perianal skin pigmentation. Surgical removal of the polyps through multiple small bowel enterotomies is necessary if symptoms due to intussusception are present. Large bowel polyps are uncommon in this disorder. There is a small increased risk of cancer in the large bowel and stomach.

Juvenile Polyposis

In juvenile polyposis it is the colon that is primarily affected and there is a small but increased risk of large bowel cancer. The polyps are easy to snare owing to the long slender stalk and should be removed by colonoscopic snare polypectomy. There is no need for major surgery in these patients. A colonoscopy should be carried out at 1-2 yearly intervals thereafter.

Familial Adenomatous Polyposis

It is now realised that the entire gastrointestinal tract may be affected in familial adenomatous polyposis. Adenomas begin to form in adolescence and rapidly increase in number. If untreated the development of large bowel cancer is certain. About two-thirds of patients presenting with symptoms (usually developing after the age of 30) already have a large bowel carcinoma. There is also an increased incidence of duodenal, periampullary and bile duct carcinoma.

Identification

There are always over 100 adenomas in the colon when the disease is fully developed and this is the essential feature which distinguishes patients with familial adenomatosis from those with sporadic adenomas, where synchronous lesions seldom exceed five in number. The diagnosis will therefore be suspected after full examination of the large bowel. Since adenomas and carcinoma may also occur in the stomach, duodenum and biliary tree, gastroduodenoscopy should be carried out as well. Some patients have tumours of connective tissues, such as fibromas, osteomas or intra-abdominal desmoids and epidermoid and odontal cysts. The association of these lesions with adenomatosis is known as Gardner's syndrome.

Removal

The method of removal differs from that described above because there is no practical way of controlling all polyps by endoscopic means. A colectomy with ileorectal anastomosis is the treatment of choice as it removes the majority of the large bowel at risk, while avoiding a stoma. The rectum can readily be kept under surveillance by regular sigmoidoscopic examination and polyps destroyed by diathermy fulguration.

Before embarking on major surgery, however, it is essential to obtain histological confirmation of adenomas. Failure to do so may result in unnecessary operations on patients with metaplastic or juvenile polyposis.

Follow-up

After colectomy and ileorectal anastomosis a regular check of the rectal stump by digital examination and sigmoidoscopy is essential. Suspicious areas of induration or ulceration should be biopsied and rectal polyps fulgurated. A 3-monthly sigmoidoscopy and a gastroduodenoscopy every 2–3 years are advisable. Despite this policy, carcinoma in the rectal stump will occur in a few patients. The incidence is low, however, and in 148 patients treated at St. Mark's Hospital over a 33-year period, only 10 (6.8%) have developed a rectal cancer and only 2 patients have subsequently died of the disease.

Patients who are anticipated to be unlikely to attend for follow-up should not be treated by ileorectal anastomosis owing to the risk of malignancy developing in the rectal stump. For these, complete removal of the large bowel mucosa is indicated. When this is necessary it is now possible to avoid an ileostomy by performing a restorative proctocolectomy with ileal reservoir.

Family History

Familial adenomatous polyposis is inherited as an autosomal dominant condition. Offspring from an affected patient have, therefore, a 50% chance of inheriting the disease. The gene is, however, rare and occurs in only about 1 in 20 000 of the population.

The aim is to identify relatives at risk either at present or in the future and a full family history should involve entering the family details on a register, construction of a family tree, identification of members at risk, and updating the register as children are born. This system will then enable those at risk to be brought to the hospital for examination, with the hope of identifying the disease before cancer has developed.

Further Reading

Bussey HJR (1975) Familial polyposis coli: Family studies, histopathology and results of treatment.
    Johns Hopkins University Press, Baltimore
Gillespie PE, Chambers TJ, Chan KW, Doronzo F, Morson BC, Williams CB (1979) Colonic
    adenomas: A colonoscopic survey. Gut 20: 240–245
Hermanek P (1983) Colorectal polyps: A precancerous condition? Internist (Berlin) 24: 71–74
Morson BC, Day D (1981) Pathology of adenomas and cancer of the large bowel. In: DeCosse JJ
    (ed) Large bowel cancer. Churchill Livingstone, Edinburgh
Morson BC, Dawson IMP (1979) Gastrointestinal pathology, 2nd edn. Blackwell Scientific, Oxford

8 Carcinoma

Carcinoma of the large bowel is the second most common malignant tumour in Western industrialised countries. In the United Kingdom there are over 20 000 new cases with 15 000 deaths reported annually, and over 100 000 new cases in the USA. It is, however, uncommon in less developed countries and in the Far East. The geographical distribution can be linked to the consumption of animal fat and protein, which may in turn be associated with alterations in the bile acid composition in faeces. Some bile acids may be co-carcinogenic and it is suggested that these may be formed by abnormal bacterial fermentation.

While epidemiological and biochemical research may be leading towards a greater understanding of the aetiology of large bowel cancer, too little is known to be of much use in practice. It is, however, apparent that there is an increased familial incidence of 3–4 times that occurring in the general population. Patients with long-standing ulcerative colitis, polyposis and schistosomiasis are at increased risk, although these three diseases account for only 1%–2% of all cases of large bowel cancer. Thus besides a positive family history there are no useful markers in the majority of cases unless the patient has previously had a large bowel carcinoma or adenoma. Then subsequent tumour formation occurs in about 5% of patients followed for 10–15 years from diagnosis of the initial neoplasm.

Carcinoma occurs predominantly in the left colon and rectum although there is some evidence to suggest that right-sided lesions are becoming more common. The incidence in the two sexes is about equal. The disease is increasingly common as age advances, but can occur in young adults even in the absence of a predisposing disease. Many large bowel cancers probably arise from malignant change within a pre-existing adenoma (see p.142). Synchronous carcinomas are found in 2%–3% of cases.

Diagnosis

Symptoms

Important symptoms include bleeding, a change in bowel habit and the passage of mucus. Altered blood mixed with the stool is highly suggestive but bleeding from a low rectal carcinoma or haemorrhoids may be indistinguishable. Sometimes, particularly with right-sided lesions, bleeding may not be noticed by the patient and the disease presents as anaemia. Left-sided colonic lesions are more likely to constrict the bowel than those in the right colon or rectum, and may give rise to obstructive symptoms including pain.

Involvement of neighbouring structures may cause pain (due to nerve invasion), ureteric obstruction, iliac vein thrombosis and fistulation to other parts of the intestine, bladder, vagina, uterus or abdominal wall. Abdominal distension may be caused by obstruction or by ascites formation as a result of peritoneal involvement. Anorexia and weight loss suggest disseminated disease but may also be due to obstruction.

Signs

The diagnosis is made on rectal digital examination, endoscopy and barium enema examination. Rigid sigmoidoscopy will identify most carcinomas of the rectum and flexible sigmoidoscopy enables most in the left colon, particularly in the sigmoid, to be diagnosed on the patient's first attendance. Blood seen in the lumen on sigmoidoscopy is an absolute indication for barium enema examination which, if normal, must be followed by colonoscopy. About 5% of carcinomas are missed on the air contrast barium enema. They are often those situated in the sigmoid colon, where diverticular disease or overlapping of barium-filled loops of bowel may obscure them. Patients with suspected colonic bleeding in whom the results of sigmoidoscopy and barium enema examination are normal must have a colonoscopy, and carcinoma will be found in 10%–20%. Whenever possible the diagnosis should be confirmed by examination of a biopsy specimen. Patients already found to have a large bowel cancer on endoscopy should have a barium enema examination to exclude a synchronous carcinoma or adenoma, unless there is a significant degree of obstruction.

Assessment (Table 8.1)

Clinical Stage

Assessment of the clinical stage preoperatively may influence the choice of operation and the decision whether to use radiotherapy in addition to surgery. In

Table 8.1. Preoperative assessment of large bowel cancer

Clinical stage	
Dissemination	General examination
	Chest X-ray
	Liver and abdominal scans
	Carcinoembryonic antigen (CEA)
Local extent	Digital examination (rectal cancer)
	± Computerised tomographic scan (CT)
	± Intravenous urogram
Histological grade	Biopsy
Synchronous tumours	Barium enema
	± Colonoscopy
Preparation for surgery	Haemoglobin
	Blood group and antibodies
	Electrocardiograph
	?Stomatherapist

some patients with advanced disease there may be no indication for specific treatment.

Dissemination

Dissemination may be apparent by the presence of liver enlargement, ascites and abdominal masses away from the site of the primary tumour, caused perhaps by deposits in the omentum or preaortic nodes. Involvement of the pelvic peritoneum may be palpable on digital examination per rectum or per vaginam. Metastases may be seen on the chest X-ray film or on isotope, ultrasonic or computerised tomographic (CT) scans of the liver. Imaging of the liver by CT may identify patients with liver secondaries which are not apparent on palpation at laparotomy (occult hepatic metastases). Preoperative detection of these lesions may in the future have an important influence on the design and outcome of clinical cancer trials.

Local Features

The clinical significance of the local features can only be appreciated on the basis of pathological stage.

PATHOLOGICAL STAGE. Prognosis is related not only to dissemination but to the local extent of the carcinoma and to the presence or absence of lymphatic or venous invasion. This can be determined accurately only by histological examination of the resected specimen. Assessment by the pathologist involves dissection of the specimen to identify nodes and veins and section of the primary tumour through the area of greatest penetration. Thus, the accuracy of the report depends on how carefully this has been done. Uncertainty over staging may mean that results from one unit cannot be compared with those of another. Furthermore, Dukes' pathological staging system has been modified in various ways so that, unfortunately, there is now no uniform standard worldwide. Although the majority of pathologists in Europe apply Dukes' system, those in the USA mostly use the modification of Astler and Coller. Both have adopted an ABC notation, but despite this confusion there is a clear relationship between stage and 5-year survival using either method (Fig. 8.1).

Pathological staging systems are really an attempt to combine two different pathological features of a tumour (penetration or not of the bowel wall and the presence or absence of lymph node metastases) into a simplified scale of indices. All have failed, however, to include two other features, namely the presence or absence of venous invasion and the extent of direct local spread within the tissues outside the bowel.

In Fig. 8.2 the influence on survival of all these pathological attributes is shown. In addition there is a relationship between local extent and the subsequent development of local recurrence (Table 8.2). It can be seen that extent of extrarectal spread is among the most important predictors of treatment failure.

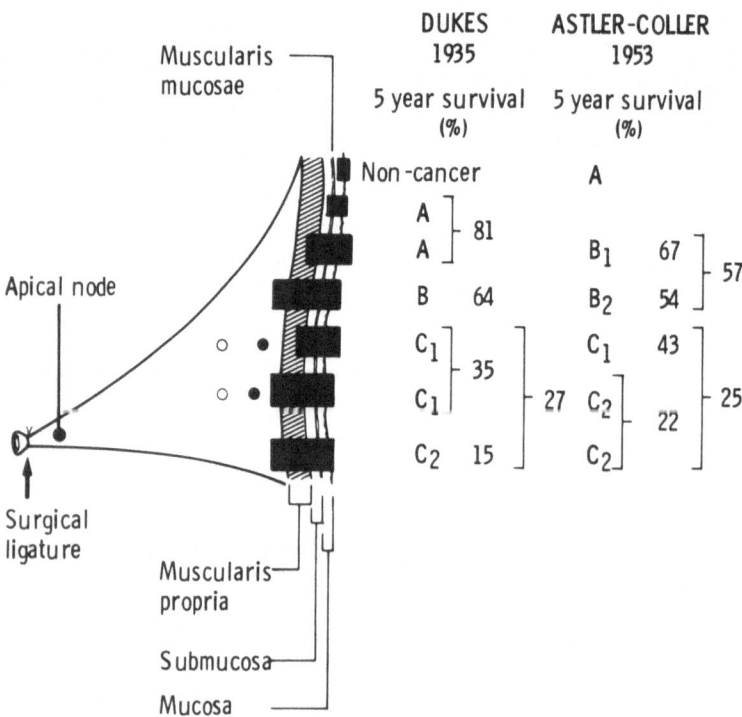

Fig. 8.1. Dukes and Astler–Coller pathological staging for cancer of the rectum, and 5-year survival (%).

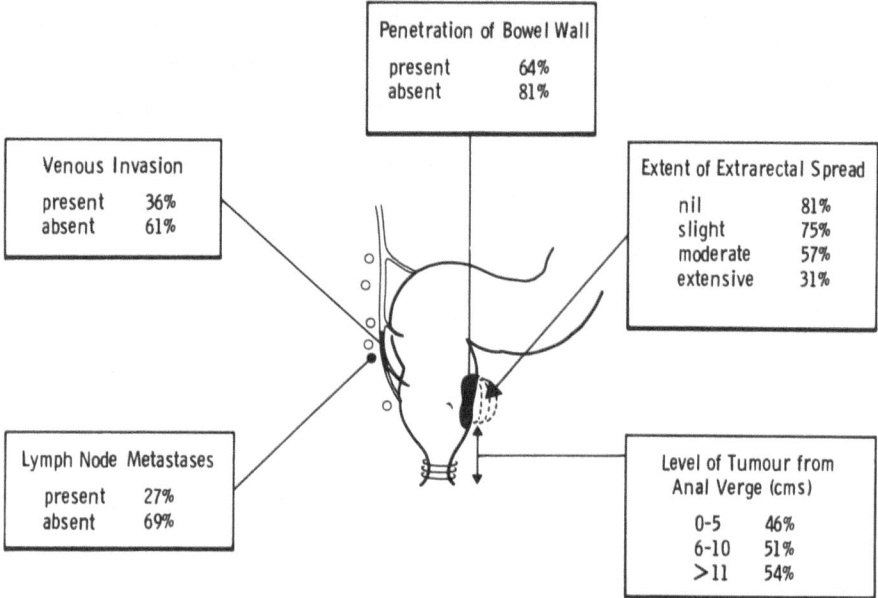

Fig. 8.2. Pathological features which influence survival; figures refer to 5-year survival rates (%) taken from several large surgical series.

Table 8.2. Rectal carcinoma: Survival and local recurrence related to degree of extrarectal spread after 'curative' surgery

	Degree of extrarectal spread		
	None	Slight	Extensive
Age-corrected survival at 5 years (%)	97	75	31
Local recurrence (%)	1	6	17

PROPOSED CLINICAL STAGING OF RECTAL CANCER. It would be helpful to have some idea of the local pathological features of a tumour preoperatively. This is particularly true with rectal cancer since there may be a choice of treatments including total rectal excision, anterior resection and local excision. A locally advanced tumour may possibly be unresectable or it may benefit from a course of preoperative radiotherapy.

While the decision depends upon clinical factors such as the age, general fitness and build of the patient and the patient's wishes, it is mostly influenced by the local pathological features. These include distance of the carcinoma from the anal verge, extent of spread into surrounding tissues, presence of local lymph node invasion and histological grade. The level of the carcinoma and histological grade can be determined by sigmoidoscopy and examination of a biopsy specimen. A very extensive carcinoma can be demonstrated by a CT scan, but local extent and lymph node involvement can in most cases only be assessed by rectal digital examination. The role of intraluminal ultrasound scanning, which has recently been used to detect local spread, is at present undefined.

Digital Examination. Most tumours up to 10–12 cm from the anal verge (i.e. in the lower two-thirds of the rectum) can be palpated, including therefore the majority for which the choice of operation has to be made. From the physical signs of mobility and the extent of tumour outside the rectum, as felt through the neighbouring normal rectal wall, it is possible to identify correctly, in about 80% of cases, tumours which are not extensive (stage 1) and those which are extensive (stage 2). A stage 1 growth is either confined to the rectal wall or has penetrated beyond to a slight degree only. In stage 2 local spread into the extrarectal tissues is extensive with the likelihood of involvement of other organs and the possibility of unresectability. Stages 1 and 2 include one subgroup each, namely stage 1A when the tumour is confined to the bowel wall and 2B where invasion of a neighbouring organ has occurred. Survival and local recurrence after surgery are related to clinical stage (Fig. 8.3).

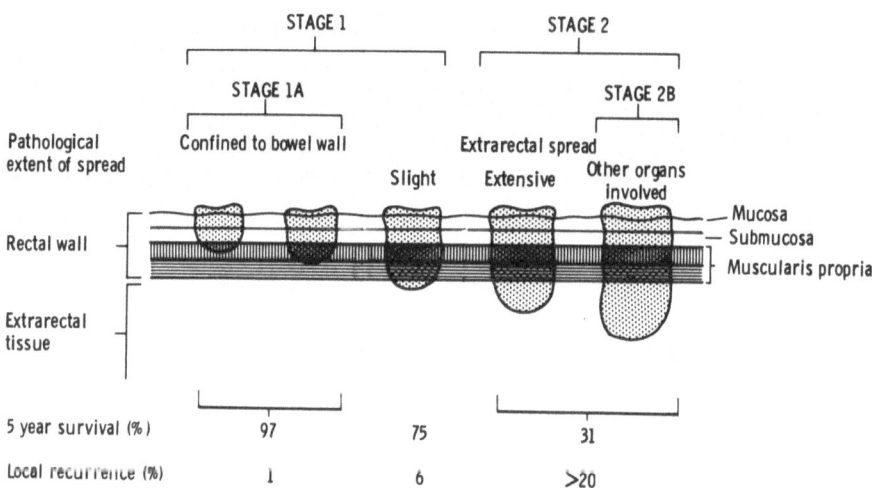

Fig. 8.3. Proposed clinical staging of cancer of the rectum; 5-year survival and local recurrence rates.

Digital examination should include an attempt to feel for enlarged lymph nodes behind the rectum. Although this is relatively inaccurate, finding nodes in a given case may be important, especially if the primary tumour might have been considered for local excision. It is a myth that the ability to palpate enlarged nodes requires specialist skill.

Management

Primary Treatment

Reported 5-year survival rates for all patients with large bowel cancer range from 20% to 40%. About 30% already have metastases on presentation and of the 70% treated by a curative procedure, about 50% will be alive at 5 years. There has been no great change in survival for several decades and no indication that chemotherapy or radiotherapy have had any influence. The latter may reduce local recurrence, but scientific proof with suitable controls is still required.

Surgery

MAJOR RESECTIONS. Surgical resection offers the best chance of cure. In the colon the strategy is straightforward, involving removal of the primary tumour with an adequate margin (approximately 5 cm) of bowel on each side of the growth and the lymphovascular pedicle as far as is anatomically possible. Any locally invaded organ should be taken en bloc.
Rectum. The rectum is a special case, however, because of the proximity of the anal sphincter.

There are many techniques for joining the colon to the rectum or anal canal and the indications for anterior resection are determined more by pathological considerations than by any shortcomings in the anastomotic methods available. The chief difference between anterior resection and total rectal excision is the extent of tissue removed distal to the tumour. Spread below its border greater than 1 cm is very uncommon provided the growth is not poorly differentiated, and a distal margin of normal rectum below the tumour of 3 cm does not appear to prejudice cure. Thus, carcinomas in the upper rectum and most in the mid rectum, i.e. more than 8 cm from the anal verge, are suitable for anterior resection.

The degree of extrarectal spread may also influence the decision, since it is inadvisable to carry out an anastomosis after removal of an extensive growth which is likely to recur locally (stage 2B), or where local clearance is known to be incomplete. Conversely, some stage 1 lesions in the upper part of the lower third of the rectum may be amenable to anterior resection without prejudicing the patient's prospect of cure.

While every reasonable effort should be made to avoid a permanent colostomy, return to acceptable bowel function after low anterior resection may take some months. In patients with liver metastases this period may exceed their life expectancy, and it is often better to carry out a total excision in such cases.
LOCAL EXCISION. Small pedunculated carcinomas may be treated by snare excision. Often carcinoma is found only after pathological examination of a specimen removed by colonoscopy. Follow-up of these cases has shown 5-year survival rates of 90% or more and unless evident tumour has been left behind further management should be expectant with check colonoscopy at 6-monthly to

yearly intervals. Patients with residual tumour as judged by colonoscopy or the demonstration by the pathologist of incomplete excision should undergo surgical resection.

With sessile carcinomas, local excision is only appropriate in a selected group of small rectal lesions where the alternative is total rectal excision with a permanent colostomy or where the patient is considered too unfit to withstand a major operation. It is not an alternative to anterior resection. It can cure carcinomas which have not spread to local lymph nodes and which are unlikely to recur locally. Selection of tumours suitable for local excision depends chiefly on two pathological factors: first the absence of penetration of the bowel wall by the carcinoma and secondly the absence of evidence indicating a high grade poorly differentiated tumour. With such growths the incidence of lymph node metastasis is less than 10% compared with 50% for those that have penetrated the rectal wall. Thus, adequate local excision should theoretically remove the tumour in about 90% of cases and this has been borne out by the clinical results.

Suitable growths for local excision are therefore those assessed as stage 1A without palpable nodes that are also small enough for complete local excision to be technically feasible (3 cm or less) and are accessible, i.e. in the lower rectum. Such carcinomas are in practice rare, comprising less than 5% of surgical series.

Pathological examination of the excised carcinoma is an integral part of management. The pathologist will be able to determine whether the preoperative clinical assessment and histological grade were correct. If they were not, removal of the rectum is indicated. With other methods of local treatment, e.g. radiotherapy and electrocoagulation, no specimen is available.

Radiotherapy

Radiotherapy is not applicable to most cases of large bowel cancer, but can be used in rectal cancer owing to the fixed position of the rectum. Used as the only primary treatment it can cure about 25% of cases, but there is a high failure rate in achieving local control (approximately 75%), particularly where the growth is extensive. Its most promising role is as an adjuvant in combination with surgery in an attempt to reduce the chance of failure of local treatment.

Used preoperatively, there is evidence that it can render an inoperable growth operable, reduce the size of the primary tumour, possibly reduce local recurrence and possibly sterilise lymph node metastases. But no clinical trial has convincingly demonstrated improved survival after preoperative adjuvant radiotherapy and those trials that suggest lowered local recurrence rates have not been satisfactorily controlled. Thus its place is at present not well defined. It should be seriously considered for patients with locally advanced tumours but its use in other cases should form part of a prospective clinical study.

There is as yet little scientific information on the value of postoperative radiotherapy owing to the lack of adequate controls and the heterogeneity of clinical groups among patients treated. Small bowel irradiation damage is a greater risk after postoperative than preoperative radiotherapy.

Chemotherapy

Chemotherapy used as an adjuvant to surgery does not improve survival, almost certainly because there is no effective drug against large bowel cancer.

Follow-up

The purpose of follow-up is fourfold: first to identify treatment failure in the hope of being able to carry out some salvage procedure, secondly to discover any missed synchronous neoplasms, thirdly to identify metachronous neoplasms and fourthly to determine survival and the disease-free interval after primary treatment. A clinical examination combined with rigid sigmoidoscopy should be performed every 6 months and a barium enema examination or colonoscopy probably carried out at 2–3-yearly intervals. The prospect of early detection of treatment failure by these methods is poor, but can be improved by monitoring serum carcinoembryonic antigen (CEA).

Treatment Failure

Metastases

Most patients with disseminated disease will die of carcinoma, although a few may live for some years, survival being related to the number of metastases present. The mean survival times of patients with multiple bilobar, multiple unilobar and solitary liver metastases are about 6, 12 and 18 months.

Surgery can offer patients with solitary and perhaps some with unilobar multiple liver metastases a prospect of long-term survival (20%–40% 5-year survival). There is a similar 5-year survival rate after resection of solitary pulmonary metastases. The difficulty in applying these salvage procedures lies in the identification of patients with suitable lesions; they comprise only about 5% of the total number of patients presenting with large bowel carcinoma. If such patients are to be identified all should be followed according to a protocol that includes frequent regular CEA estimations and body scanning: a costly undertaking.

The role of chemotherapy in advanced disease has been extensively studied. Partial clinical response occurs in about 20% of patients treated with 5-fluorouracil and in 15% of those treated with methyl CCNU and mitomycin C, but there is no evidence that survival among responders is prolonged when compared with that of patients who have not been treated at all. There is therefore little indication for the use of cytotoxic drugs unless it is believed that pain is due to metastases, when regression may lead to relief, or where drug treatment is part of a scientific clinical trial.

Local Recurrence

Local recurrence occurs in up to 50% of patients undergoing primary resection of large bowel cancer and is related to the local extent of the original tumour. Although responsible for a great deal of morbidity, it is less important than disseminated disease as a cause of death. In a detailed epidemiological study from Malmö, Sweden, only 8% of patients with local recurrence did not have coexisting disease at post-mortem. The majority of local recurrences (80%) appear within 2 years of primary treatment. It is important wherever possible to confirm the diagnosis by histological examination, if necessary by needle biopsy under anaesthetic. Only in this way can data be relied upon.

Local recurrence may present as a mass or through the effects of local infiltration (for example pain, obstruction or fistulation). Pelvic recurrence in males after total rectal excision may be very difficult to diagnose and a CT scan is often helpful. In females the lower pelvis can be assessed by vaginal examination.

Attempts have been made to resect local recurrence and there is now a considerable body of data on the results of surgery used either where recurrence is clinically detected or when applied as a 'second look' strategy. Only about 10%–15% of local recurrences are apparently completely resectable and only about 10% of these patients survive for more than 2 years. This salvage rate of less than 5% is similar to the operative mortality rate for these procedures.

It is argued that these poor results might be improved if recurrence were detected before clinical presentation. Monitoring of the serum CEA has been shown to anticipate clinical recurrence sometimes by several months. There is some preliminary evidence suggesting that operations prompted by a raised CEA titre may have a greater prospect of resecting all apparent tumour, but further reports are required before this can be confirmed. Often the CEA level is not raised when local recurrence predominates over disseminated disease.

Symptoms from local pelvic recurrence such as pain or bleeding may be improved by radiotherapy, but there is little prospect of long-term survival. In some cases a symptomatic response may be sustained for a few weeks to months only.

Further Reading

Alexander-Williams J (1982) Assessing the problem, preparing the patient and minimising the risks in rectal cancer surgery. World J Surg 6: 510–516

Astler VA, Coller FA (1954) The prognostic significance of direct extension of carcinoma of the colon and rectum. Ann Surg 139: 846–852

Beart RW, O'Connell MJ (1983) Post-operative follow-up of patients with carcinoma of the colon. Mayo Clin Proc 58: 361–363

Berge T, Ekelund G, Mellner C, Pihl B, Wenkert A (1973) Carcinoma of the colon and rectum in a defined population. Acta Chir Scand [Suppl] 438

Cummings BJ, Rider WD, Harwood AR, Keane TJ, Thomas GM (1983) Radical external beam radiation therapy for adenocarcinoma. Dis Colon Rectum 26: 30–36

Davis NC, Newland RC (1983) Terminology and classification of colorectal adenocarcinoma. The Australian clinico-pathological staging system. Aust NZ J Surg 53: 211–221

Donegan WL, DeCosse JJ (1978) Pitfalls and controversies in the staging of colorectal carcinoma. In: Enker WE (ed) Carcinoma of the colon and rectum. Year Book Medical Publishers, Chicago, pp 40–70

Dukes CE, Bussey HJR (1958) The spread of rectal cancer and its effect on prognosis. Br J Cancer 12: 309–320

Enker WE (ed) (1978) Carcinoma of the colon and rectum. Year Book Medical Publishers, Chicago

Finlay IG, McArdle CS (1982) The identification of patients at high risk following curative resection for colorectal carcinoma. Br J Surg 69: 513–519

Gilbert JM (1982) Adjuvant chemotherapy of large bowel cancer. Cancer Treat Rep 9: 195–228

Hager T, Gall FB, Hermanek P (1983) Local excision of cancer of the rectum. Dis Colon Rectum 26: 149–151

Hardcastle JD (1982) Colorectal cancer. Early diagnosis and detection. Recent Results Cancer Res 83: 86–100

Hill MJ (1981) Metabolic epidemiology of large bowel cancer. In: DeCosse J and Sherlock P (ed) Gastrointestinal cancer. Martinus Nijhoff, The Hague, pp 187–226

James RD Johnson RJ, Eddeston B, Zheng GL, Jones JM (1983) Prognostic factors in locally recurrent rectal carcinoma treated by radiotherapy. Br J Surg 70: 469–472

Muto T, Bussey HJR, Morson BC (1975) The evolution of cancer of the colon and rectum. Cancer 36: 2251–2270

Nicholls RJ (1982) Colorectal cancer: Surgery. Recent Results Cancer Res 83: 101–112

Nicholls RJ, Mason AY, Morson BC, Dixon AK, Fry IK (1982) The clinical staging of rectal carcinoma. Br J Surg 69: 404–409

Nivatvongs S, Gilbertsen VA, Goldberg SM, Williams SE (1982) Distribution of large-bowel cancers detected by occult blood test in asymptomatic patients. Dis Colon Rectum 25: 420–421

Stubbs RS (1983) The aetiology of colorectal cancer. Br J Surg 70: 313–316

Weakley FL (1983) Cancer of the rectum: A review of surgical options. Surg Clin North Am 63 (1): 129–135

Wynder EL (1975) The epidemiology of large bowel cancer. Cancer Res 35: 3388–3394

9 Inflammatory Bowel Disease

There are many causes of inflammatory bowel disease (Table 9.1). In Western industrialised countries inflammation is due mainly to ulcerative colitis or Crohn's disease, but these are rare in the tropics and Mediterranean countries where the majority of cases are due to infection such as amoebiasis or bacillary dysentery.

Table 9.1. Types of inflammatory bowel disease

Idiopathic	Ulcerative colitis
	Crohn's disease
Infective	Bacillary dysentery: *Shigella, Salmonella*
	Amoebic colitis
	Schistosomiasis
	Campylobacter proctocolitis
	Pseudomembranous colitis
	Sexually transmitted diseases
	Tuberculosis
	Worms
Traumatic	Rectal prolapse
	Solitary ulcer
	Instrumentation
Ischaemic	Ischaemic colitis
Radiation	Enteritis
	Proctocolitis
Drugs	Purgatives
	Antibiotic associated

The final diagnosis can often only be made by combining clinical, radiological and bacteriological information with histopathological findings. Specific histological features (such as the presence of granulomata in Crohn's disease) may be found on examining biopsy or surgical specimens, but the colon appears to have a limited pattern of response to an inflammatory stimulus and considerable overlap of signs may exist. The aetiology of ulcerative colitis and Crohn's disease is unknown.

Diagnosis

Symptoms

The patient usually complains of diarrhoea, often with blood and mucus, and there may be systemic symptoms of weight loss, anorexia and anaemia. Occasionally, patients with ulcerative colitis or Crohn's disease may be constipated. The severity of symptoms is an indication of the severity of the disease.

The history may suggest an infective cause—for example the patient may have been in contact with a case of diarrhoea or have recently visited a country where infective colitis is endemic. There may be a past history of irradiation to the abdomen or pelvis; the latency between radiotherapy and the clinical onset of radiation enteritis can be many years. A positive family history is found in about 5%–10% of patients with ulcerative colitis and Crohn's disease. A list of drugs taken by the patient must be made, with particular reference to recent antibiotic treatment and aperients.

Signs

In most cases of inflammatory bowel disease there are no general or abdominal physical signs. However, patients with severe disease may have electrolyte depletion, malnutrition, toxicity, and extra-alimentary lesions (see below). In some cases of Crohn's disease, an abdominal mass or fistula may be present and anal lesions are common.

Inflammatory bowel disease most usually comes to light on sigmoidoscopy and further investigation of the large bowel. Cases can be divided into those with proctitis and those without. The steps involved in making a diagnosis in patients with proctitis are shown in Table 9.2.

Proctitis Present

Sometimes it is difficult on sigmoidoscopy to be sure that the rectal mucosa is inflamed. The most sensitive sign is loss of the normal vascular pattern as a result

Table 9.2. Procedure in patients with proctitis

1. History and general examination

2. Sigmoidoscopy (rigid ± flexible)
   Identify proctitis
   Appearances: ?patchy or diffuse
   Determine proximal extent

3. Microbiology
   Stool
   Rectal swab
   ± Vaginal and urethral swabs

4. Radiology
   Patient systemically ill
   Admit to hospital
   Plain abdominal X-ray film
   ? colonic dilatation
   Patient not systemically ill
   Proximal limit of disease not determined by sigmoidoscopy:
   Instant barium enema
   Proximal limit determined but further disease still suspected:
   Barium enema with full bowel preparation
   Barium follow-through

5. Histology: rectal biopsy

of mucosal oedema, but with more severe inflammation, mucosal erythema, contact bleeding, ulceration and pus or mucus in the lumen are seen. Fine granularity indicates acute inflammation while coarse granularity is a manifestation of chronic disease where previous repair and mucosal regeneration have occurred.

It is important to note the distribution of the inflammation. Continuous disease starting in the upper anal canal and spreading proximally suggests ulcerative colitis whereas patchy disease with intervening areas of normal mucosa is more likely to be found in Crohn's disease. Gonococcal proctitis is characterised by the presence of a purulent exudate adherent to the mucosa with little by way of mucosal erythema or bleeding; inflammation rarely extends beyond the lower rectum. Infective colitis caused by *Campylobacter* or *Entamoeba histolytica* may be indistinguishable from ulcerative colitis.

INVESTIGATION. Having identified the presence of proctitis, the anatomical extent of inflammation and the precise pathological diagnosis should be determined.

Extent of Disease. In patients with inflammation confined to the rectum and lower sigmoid, it is usually possible to determine the extent by rigid sigmoidoscopy. Flexible sigmoidoscopy is useful in assessing more extensive disease in the left side of the colon, but contrast radiology has the advantages of being both a complete examination of the colon and a permanent record. The choice must be made between an instant barium enema with no bowel preparation and a barium enema after full bowel preparation. The former is suitable where there is continuous disease from the rectum upwards (as in ulcerative colitis), whereas the latter should be requested where inflammation is patchy (as in Crohn's disease) and there is the likelihood of intervening segments of normal bowel containing faeces. Barium enema is contraindicated in severely ill patients, especially those with colonic dilation. A small bowel meal is required in patients with Crohn's disease.

Pathological Diagnosis. A stool sample should be sent for microbiological examination in every case of proctitis. Where amoebiasis is suspected this should be examined within 3–4 hours. In gonococcal proctitis, rectal, urethral and high vaginal swabs should be taken.

A biopsy of inflamed mucosa is essential. Radiologists are unwilling to perform a barium enema examination within 10 days of a biopsy. Accordingly a patient suitable for an instant barium enema should have the X-ray first.

Proctitis Absent

Where there is no rectal inflammation the problem is to distinguish proximal inflammatory bowel disease from other diseases which can produce similar symptoms. In the colon these include tumours, ischaemic and radiation colitis, diverticular and functional bowel disease and in the small bowel and pancreas tumours, radiation enteritis and malabsorption. General medical diseases such as thyrotoxicosis or diabetes mellitus can produce a similar clinical picture to inflammatory bowel disease and many drugs cause diarrhoea. Psychiatric disturbances such as anorexia nervosa and anxiety occasionally present with symptoms suggesting colitis.

Barium enema examination should be carried out after full preparation of the colon, followed by a small bowel meal if the results of the enema are normal. When Crohn's disease is suspected a rectal biopsy should be taken even when the rectum appears normal, since microscopic inflammation may be present. Colonoscopy is indicated where a colonic cause has not been excluded by radiological examination or if a biopsy is required. Investigation of absorptive function may be needed.

Assessment of Severity

Having made the diagnosis of inflammatory bowel disease, the severity should be determined in order to select the appropriate treatment. Severity is gauged from an assessment of the following:

Extent of disease
Severity of symptoms
Nutrition and growth
Extra-alimentary disease
Haemoglobin and blood indices
Water and electrolyte balance

Signs of toxicity
Abdominal tenderness and distension
Anal disease (Crohn's disease)

The extent of colonic disease is determined by endoscopy and radiology, which will have been carried out in making the diagnosis. Symptoms may be divided into those pertaining to the bowel, for example frequency of defaecation, urgency, blood loss and abdominal pain, and those indicating systemic disturbance, which include anorexia, weight loss, lassitude and other features of anaemia or malnutrition. Nutrition and growth can be assessed from the body weight and height (relating them to age in the case of a child), and skinfold thickness as an indirect indication of lean body mass. The presence of extra-alimentary disorders indicates severe disease; some resolve with remission, others do not (Table 9.3).

Table 9.3. Non-infective inflammatory bowel disease: Extra-alimentary manifestations

Site	Prevalence in severe disease	Manifestation
Joints	~20%	Sacroiliitis (ankylosing spondylitis) Seronegative polyarthropathy[a]

Liver	5%–10% abnormal liver function tests	Parenchymal liver disease:
		  minor histological abnormalities
		  active chronic hepatitis
		  cirrhosis
		  ($\pm$ portal hypertension)
		Sclerosing cholangitis
		Gallstones
		Bile duct carcinoma

Skin	~5%	Pyoderma gangrenosum[a]
		  (ulcerative colitis)
		Erythema nodosum[a]
		  (Crohn's disease)

	~20%	Clubbing (esp. Crohn's disease)
Eyes	~5%	Anterior uveitis[a] Episcleritis[a]
Oral cavity	20%–30%	Aphthous ulceration[a]
Lungs	Unknown	? Bronchiectasis ? Autoimmune lung disease

[a] Related to activity of disease.

Ulcerative colitis and Crohn's colitis have a natural tendency to exacerbations and remissions. The frequency and severity of relapses and the degree of disability in patients with chronic disease are therefore important factors in assessing severity. These are best judged by fitness for normal activity such as work, sport etc., and by the need for hospitalisation.

Clinical Classification

Severity can be classified as mild, moderate or severe (Table 9.4). Patients with mild or moderate disease can usually be treated medically as outpatients. Those with severe disease, particularly if suffering from an acute exacerbation, will require admission to hospital and some will need surgery.

Table 9.4. Non-infective inflammatory bowel disease: Clinical classification of severity

	Mild	Moderate	Severe
Extent	Localised	Intermediate degree of involvement	Most of large bowel involved
(Ulcerative colitis)	(Rectum)	(Rectum and sigmoid)	(Transverse colon and more proximal)
Symptoms			
Local	+	+ +	+ +
General	−	−	+
Extra-alimentary manifestations	−	−	±
Malnutrition including anaemia, retardation of growth	−	−	+
Toxicity, water and electrolyte depletion	−	−	+

Acute Severe Colitis

About 5%-10% of patients with ulcerative colitis and colonic Crohn's disease present with acute severe disease. It is important to recognise these cases since there is an appreciable mortality if treatment is delayed. Illness is due to three factors: malnutrition, water and electrolyte depletion and toxaemia. Loss of protein in the stool combined with poor food intake results in negative nitrogen balance. Water, sodium and potassium losses through diarrhoea lead to hypovolaemia and electrolyte disturbances, ultimately causing circulatory failure. Breakdown of the colonic mucosal barrier may result in septicaemia and as the disease progresses the colon can become grossly dilated (toxic dilatation) with the risk of perforation and peritonitis.

Patients with acute severe colitis have severe symptoms which include excessive frequency of defaecation (for example > 10 times per 24 hours), blood persistently in the stool, weight loss greater than 10% of normal body weight and abdominal tenderness. Anaemia, hypoalbuminaemia, tachycardia and signs of water and sodium depletion may be present and extra-alimentary lesions are often seen. The colon is usually extensively involved.

Toxic Dilatation

Toxic dilatation causes abdominal distension and is usually accompanied by pyrexia and abdominal tenderness, though not always, especially if the patient has been taking high doses of steroids. Distension is best demonstrated by a plain X-ray film of the abdomen and is defined by a colonic diameter of more than 6 cm. Other radiological signs include absence of faecal shadowing in the caecum, thickened bowel wall and circumscribed shadowing indicating the presence of oedematous mucosal islands.

Non-infective Inflammatory Bowel Disease

Ulcerative colitis and Crohn's disease occur throughout the world and among all races, but both are very much more common in Caucasians living in Europe and North America. Ulcerative colitis occurs with equal frequency in both sexes, but Crohn's disease is more common in females. The incidence of Crohn's disease appears to be increasing whereas that of ulcerative colitis is stable.

The aetiology is unknown, but there is an increased familial incidence of both diseases among already affected close relatives. No specific pathogen has been isolated and no possibly causative immunological disorder has been found. Some patients do show abnormalities of immune reactivity but these are probably related to the severity of illness rather than to the disease itself. There is a suggestion that Crohn's disease may be associated with the long-term ingestion of refined foods, but further information is required to validate this contention.

Ulcerative Colitis or Crohn's Disease?

The clinical and radiological characteristics of ulcerative colitis and Crohn's disease are a reflection of different pathology and their contrasting features are summarised in Table 9.5. The essential differences are the extent of the gastro-

Table 9.5. Main pathological differences between Crohn's disease and ulcerative colitis

	Crohn's disease	Ulcerative colitis
General pathological features	Entire alimentary tract at risk	Colon only
	Focal (patchy)	Diffuse
	Full thickness involvement of bowel wall	Confined to mucosa
Rectum	Often spared	Almost always involved
Anal disease	Common	Uncommon

intestinal tract that is susceptible, the patchy distribution of Crohn's disease compared with the diffuse involvement of ulcerative colitis, and the full thickness inflammation of bowel in Crohn's disease in contrast to the mucosal involvement of ulcerative colitis. Patchiness is a very important sign that can be seen radiologically, endoscopically and histologically. Indeed, it is the most useful criterion for the pathologist when examining a biopsy specimen. If a microscopic area of relatively normal crypt glands is seen next to inflamed crypts, Crohn's disease is more likely. The presence of intervening microscopic or macroscopic normal tissue between areas of inflammation is the cardinal sign of Crohn's disease. Certain other histological features may also help in diagnosis, as shown in Figs. 9.1 and 9.2.

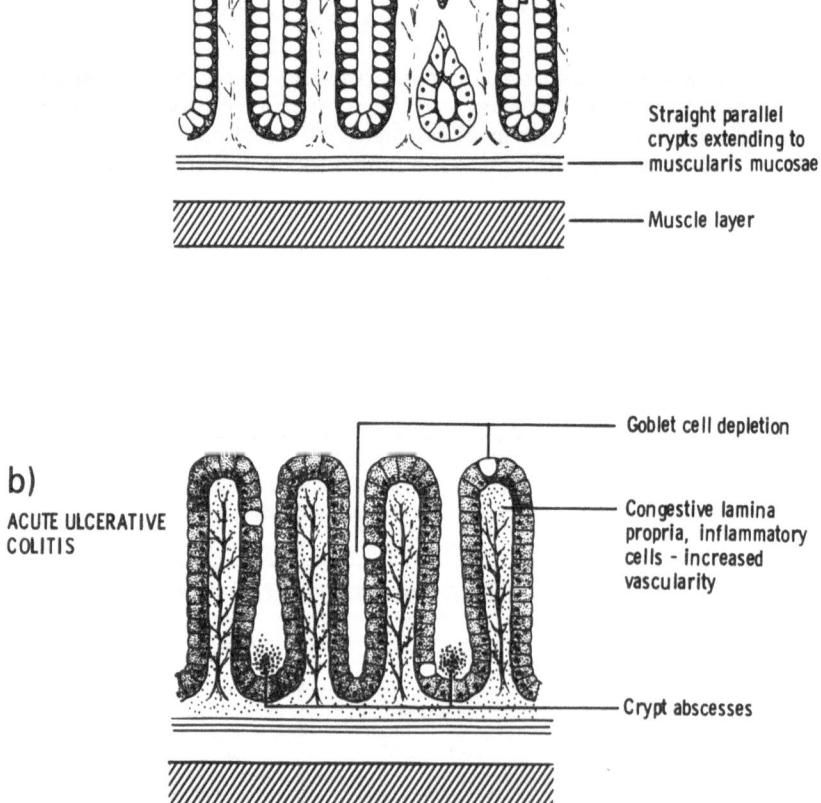

a)

NORMAL

Goblet cell filled
with mucus

Straight parallel
crypts extending to
muscularis mucosae

Muscle layer

b)

ACUTE ULCERATIVE
COLITIS

Goblet cell depletion

Congestive lamina
propria, inflammatory
cells - increased
vascularity

Crypt abscesses

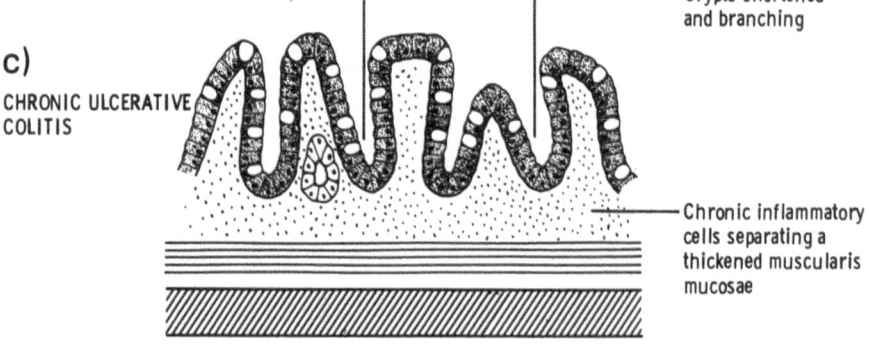

c)

CHRONIC ULCERATIVE
COLITIS

Crypts shortened
and branching

Chronic inflammatory
cells separating a
thickened muscularis
mucosae

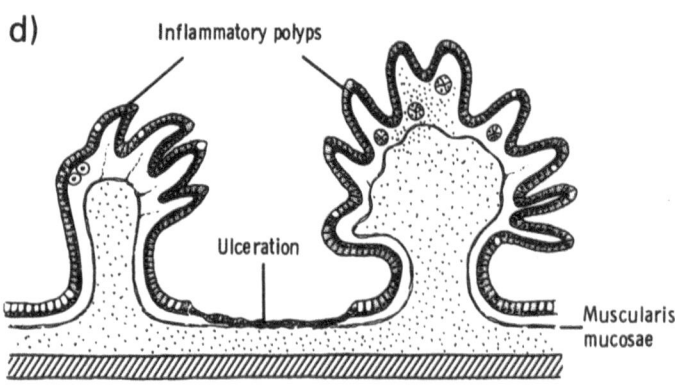

d)

Inflammatory polyps

Ulceration

Muscularis
mucosae

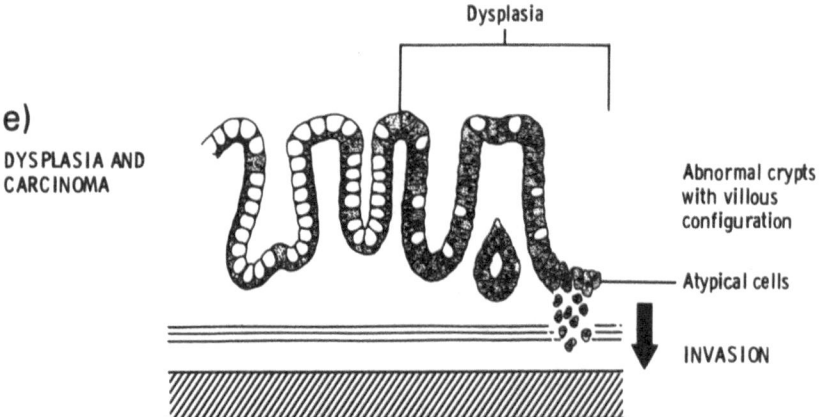

e)

DYSPLASIA AND
CARCINOMA

Dysplasia

Abnormal crypts
with villous
configuration

Atypical cells

INVASION

Fig. 9.1a–e. Histological changes in ulcerative colitis.

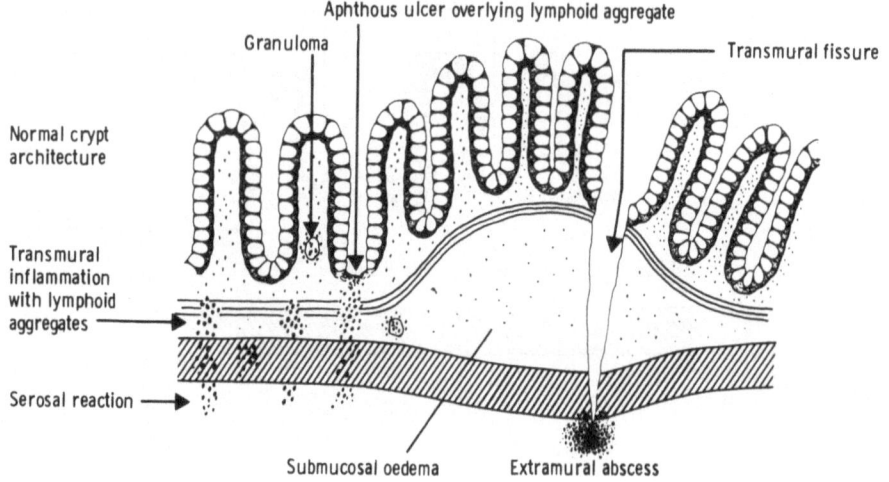

Fig. 9.2. Histological changes in Crohn's disease.

The rectum is almost always affected in ulcerative colitis whereas rectal inflammation is present in only about 50% of patients with Crohn's colitis. In ulcerative colitis the disease seems to spread from the distal to the proximal bowel; the proportions of patients with different degrees of involvement at presentation are shown in Fig. 9.3.

In Crohn's disease transmural involvement leads to fibrosis with stricture formation and obstruction. Ulceration penetrates the bowel wall forming fissures which deepen to the serosa; this in turn produces a local peritoneal reaction causing peri-intestinal abscess formation with fistulation into adherent structures on spontaneous rupture or surgical drainage.

About one-third of patients presenting with Crohn's disease have colonic involvement, the symptoms of which are indistinguishable from those of ulcerative colitis. In about 15% of cases of non-infective colitis it is impossible to decide between the two possible diagnoses. Usually, however, the diagnosis becomes apparent with time and more often turns out to be Crohn's disease. Patients with anal disease, erythema nodosum, finger nail clubbing and oral aphthous ulceration are more likely to have Crohn's disease.

Two-thirds of patients with Crohn's disease present with small bowel involvement. In 20% of all cases inflammation appears to be confined to the small bowel, but in 40% or more the terminal ileum and the right side of the colon are both affected. The pathological process leading to stricture and abscess formation produces a different clinical picture to that seen in cases of colitis. Intestinal obstruction (usually chronic) and abscess and fistula formation are the commonest forms of clinical presentation in small intestinal or ileocaecal Crohn's disease.

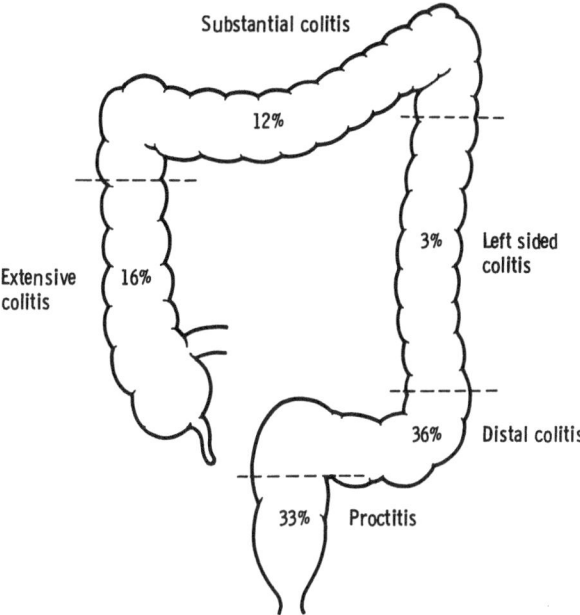

Fig. 9.3. The extent of ulcerative colitis on presentation (% of cases).

Management

About 80% of patients with ulcerative colitis can be treated without surgery, whereas 80% of those with Crohns disease will require an operation at some time during the course of the disease. Management can be divided into treatment of colitis and the treatment of Crohn's disease affecting parts of the gastrointestinal tract other than the large bowel. A more detailed description will be found in textbooks of gastroenterology and surgery. Close co-operation between physician and surgeon is often the key to making the correct decision at the right time.

Colitis (Table 9.6)

Medical Treatment

Mild and moderate colitis and many cases of severe disease can be managed by medical means. Medical treatment of ulcerative colitis and Crohn's colitis is the same and can be divided into anti-inflammatory agents, symptomatic treatment, replacement therapy and dietary measures.

ANTI-INFLAMMATORY AGENTS. The aims of anti-inflammatory treatment are first to induce and then to maintain a remission. Anti-inflammatory drugs

Table 9.6. Non-infective inflammatory bowel disease: Summary of treatment

	Outpatient	Admission to hospital	Operation
Proctitis alone	Local steroids Sulphasalazine	–	–
Left-sided colitis	Local steroids Sulphasalazine ± Antidiarrhoeals ± Iron replacement	Occasionally necessary	Rare
Extensive colitis	Systemic steroids (oral) Sulphasalazine Antidiarrhoeals Iron Nutrition	May be necessary	May be necessary (elective)

Acute severe colitis	–	*Admit*
		Systemic steroids
		  (intravenous)
		Water and electrolyte
		  replacement
		Nutrition (? intravenous)
		± Blood transfusion
			Often necessary
			(semi-urgent)

Toxic dilatation	–	*Admit* Resuscitation	Obligatory (urgent)

include corticosteroids, sulphasalazine (Salazopyrin) and azathioprine. There is no evidence that antibiotics influence the inflammatory process in colitis. Sodium cromoglycate has not been shown to be effective.

Corticosteroids. Corticosteroids induce remission of disease. They can be given systemically or topically by suppository or enema, depending on the site and extent of inflammation. In distal proctitis prednisolone suppositories (5 mg) may be all that is needed, but if the disease extends proximally to the upper rectum and sigmoid colon, enemas should be given. Proprietary preparations (Predsol, Colifoam) are available but some physicians recommend that the patient prepares his own enemas, dissolving prednisolone 21-phosphate (10–40 mg) in 50–100 ml of tapwater. Suppositories or enemas should be given at night and the dose adjusted according to the extent and severity of disease.

Patients with extensive colitis or systemic symptoms should be given oral prednisolone, initially in a dose of 30–60 mg daily. Severely ill patients with acute colitis require admission to hospital and should be treated by intravenous prednisolone. Whenever possible, steroid treatment should be reduced and finally stopped after remission has occurred. In some cases, however, it is necessary to leave the patient on maintenance treatment.

Sulphasalazine. Sulphasalazine has been shown to be effective in maintaining remission in ulcerative colitis but is of less certain value in Crohn's disease. It is a bonded combination of sulphapyridine and 5-amino salicylic acid which is broken down into its constituents by bacterial enzymic action in the large bowel. Evidence suggests that salicylic acid is the active agent.

The dose is 2–4 g per day in divided doses; the nausea and indigestion which some patients experience may be avoided by prescribing the more expensive enteric coated tablets. Other unwanted effects include skin rashes and blood dyscrasia. Side effects are mostly due to the sulphonamide moiety. Sulphasalazine is given with corticosteroids at the start of treatment and continued indefinitely after remission. It is not known for how long treatment should be maintained.

Azathioprine. Some clinical trials have indicated that azathioprine given to patients with Crohn's disease may reduce the chance of further surgery being required. When continued for months, it appears to have an anti-inflammatory effect and allows the maintenance dose of steroids to be reduced. It can, however, cause sudden and severe depression of the bone marrow and careful monitoring by monthly blood counts is obligatory. Its use should be confined to patients with severe Crohn's disease who have already had resection and for whom steroids do not seem to be helping.

SYMPTOMATIC TREATMENT. Drugs may be needed to control diarrhoea. Loperamide (Imodium) and codeine phosphate are effective. Long-term administration may be necessary and there is a danger of codeine dependence.

REPLACEMENT THERAPY. Patients with iron-deficiency anaemia require iron medication. Vitamin B12 malabsorption and folate deficiency may follow resection or increased bacterial colonisation of the small bowel.

DIETARY MEASURES. A normal diet should be recommended, with modifications under three circumstances. Some colitics (about 5%) have lactase deficiency and should avoid milk and milk products. Patients with stricture formation should avoid foods liable to cause bolus obstruction—for example skins of sausages or tomatoes or the fibrous parts of fruits and vegetables. Small bowel disease in some patients with Crohn's disease occasionally causes malabsorption, and in such cases a low-fat diet may help to reduce diarrhoea. The suggestion that a high-fibre diet reduces the likelihood of recurrence of Crohn's disease is non-proven.

ACUTE SEVERE COLITIS. Patients with acute severe colitis should be admitted to hospital and water and electrolyte depletion corrected by intravenous infusion. Blood transfusion may be necessary if there is severe anaemia. Steroids are indicated and should be given intravenously. The patient is carefully monitored for signs of improvement, particular attention being paid to the pulse, temperature and abdominal signs including tenderness and dilatation. A plain abdominal X-ray film will enable the degree of colonic distension to be assessed. Surgery is indicated if improvement does not occur within a few days or if colonic dilatation develops.

Surgery

Surgery may be indicated as an emergency or it may be elective (Table 9.7); with few exceptions it is necessary only for patients with extensive involvement of the large bowel.

EMERGENCY. Emergency indications are easy to define and while the timing depends on the condition of the patient it is better to intervene earlier rather than

Table 9.7. Non-infective colitis: Indications for surgery

Emergency	Toxic dilatation
	Bleeding (rare)
Elective	Failed medical treatment
	Acute attack; failure to resolve
	Recurrent exacerbations
	Chronic ill-health
	Uncontrolled symptoms
	Retardation of growth
	Carcinoma/dysplasia
	Anal disease (Crohn's disease)

later. The operation of choice is colectomy and terminal ileostomy with preservation of the rectum. This procedure carries a lower mortality than emergency total proctocolectomy and a decision as to further management of the rectal stump can be deferred until a later date. Surgery is indicated as a semi-emergency in cases of acute severe colitis which fail to respond to initial intensive medical treatment.

ELECTIVE. Assessment of patients with chronic disease for surgery requires experience and familiarity with the patient's individual circumstances and temperament. Anal disease as a reason for surgery almost exclusively applies to Crohn's disease.

Ulcerative Colitis. There are three operations available for ulcerative colitis, namely total proctocolectomy, colectomy and ileorectal anastomosis and restorative proctocolectomy with ileal reservoir and ileoanal anastomosis. Partial colectomy is unsatisfactory owing to the likelihood of recurrence in the remaining colon. Total proctocolectomy is curative since all disease tissue is excised, but the patient is left with a permanent ileostomy. Colectomy with ileorectal anastomosis avoids an ileostomy but recurrent inflammation or the development of malignant change in the rectum is responsible for failure (i.e. subsequent excision of the rectum and conversion to a permanent ileostomy) in 25%–35% of cases. With restorative proctocolectomy with ileal reservoir the entire large bowel mucosa is removed without an ileostomy while preserving satisfactory bowel function in most cases.

Colectomy with ileorectal anastomosis is excluded in patients with severe rectal inflammation or rectal narrowing and where severe dysplasia or frank malignancy is already present. The choice between total and restorative proctocolectomy depends on the wishes of the patient—provided Crohn's disease has been excluded and the patient is fully aware of the longer period of treatment required and the possible complications (including a failure rate of 5%–10%) that may occur after restorative proctocolectomy.

Crohn's Colitis. The choice of operation in Crohn's colitis depends on the extent and location of the disease. A limited area can be treated by segmental resection although if severe inflammation involves the rectum or anal region a rectal excision will be necessary. Extensive large bowel involvement should be treated by total proctocolectomy. Ileorectal anastomosis is indicated where there is rectal sparing or mild rectal inflammation only. Restorative proctocolectomy with ileal reservoir is contraindicated in Crohn's disease. The management of anal Crohn's disease is discussed on p.106.

Unlike surgery for ulcerative colitis, that for Crohn's disease is not curative and is often followed by recurrence, usually in the terminal ileum, which in many cases requires further surgery. The recurrence rate over a 5-year period is 50% after segmental resection or ileorectal anastomosis. It is significantly less, however, where a stoma has been created (10%–30%).

The Cancer Risk

The risk of cancer is considerably greater in ulcerative colitis than in Crohn's disease and is confined almost entirely to cases of extensive disease. In practice, these include patients with an intact large bowel being managed medically and those who have undergone colectomy with ileorectal anastomosis. In the former group the entire colon is at risk while in the latter only the rectum is susceptible. The incidence of cancer is related to the duration and not to age of onset of the disease.

In ulcerative colitis the cumulative risk over a 20-year period is about 5%–10% with a steady rise thereafter. It is negligible within 10 years of diagnosis, after which time patients must be monitored by regular (6-monthly) endoscopy and biopsy. Where the entire colon is intact colonoscopy is necessary, but rigid sigmoidoscopy only is sufficient after colectomy with ileorectal anastomosis.

Although frank carcinoma may be found, a premalignant state (severe dysplasia) can also be recognised by the pathologist (Fig. 9.1e). The finding of severe dysplasia on two successive occasions (e.g. two outpatient visits at 6-monthly intervals) is an indication for surgery since it implies impending malignant transformation.

Small Bowel Crohn's Disease

As in the large bowel, surgery will not cure Crohn's disease and should be looked upon as a means of dealing with a localised complication. In practice indications for surgery in small bowel Crohn's disease include intestinal obstruction and fistula or abscess formation. An acute abscess pointing to the exterior should be drained, but in most cases this results in an enterocutaneous fistula which will require subsequent resection. Recurrence after segmental resection of small bowel or ileocaecal Crohn's disease is common, with re-operation rates over a 5–10-year follow-up period of about 50%–80%. Extensive resection of small bowel has been claimed by some surgeons to reduce recurrence rates, but no clinical trial of extensive versus limited resection has been reported. Radical surgery has the real disadvantage of increasing the chance of producing a short bowel syndrome without having any obvious long-term advantage of control of the disease.

Infective Inflammatory Bowel Disease

Bacillary Dysentery

Bacillary dysentery is a highly contagious disease caused by organisms of the genus *Shigella*. The bacteria are confined to the gastrointestinal tract and excreted in high concentrations in the faeces. The whole colon is affected and rapidly becomes oedematous with areas of haemorrhage. Necrosis of the epithelium can occur with the formation of a membrane.

Clinical Features

The incubation period is 1–7 days. The patient then develops a high fever, abdominal colic and watery blood-stained diarrhoea. The attack may be accompanied by an arthropathy and inflammatory eye lesions. It is easy to see how the clinical picture can be confused with ulcerative colitis or Crohn's disease. There is, however, often a history of contact, travel to areas where bacillary dysentery is endemic or a definable local epidemic of the disease. The final diagnosis is made on the isolation of the causative organism in the stool.

Treatment

In severe cases replacement of lost water and electrolytes is needed. Usually this can be accomplished by mouth but intravenous administration may be necessary, particularly in young children.

Unless the illness is so severe that immediate treatment is demanded, antibiotics should be reserved until the causative organism has been isolated. The organism is sensitive to non-absorbable sulphonamides or oral tetracycline. Ampicillin and chloramphenicol are also effective and the choice of antibiotic must be related to the sensitivity of the causative organism.

Amoebic Colitis

Infection by cysts of the protozoon *Entamoeba histolytica* occurs via ingestion of contaminated food and drink. The cyst wall is destroyed by gastrointestinal enzymes, releasing the active amoebae to invade the mucosa and submucosa. There they produce superficial and deeper ulcers which develop secondary bacterial infection. Amoebae may enter the portal venous circulation and travel to the liver to produce an amoebic liver abscess.

Clinical Features

After an incubation period of 7–10 days the patient develops severe bloody diarrhoea leading to dehydration and electrolyte depletion. The attack may settle after some days or it may persist and sometimes progress to toxic dilatation, which is usually lethal. The disease may recur in cases where resolution has taken place to become chronic amoebic dysentery, causing intermittent attacks of diarrhoea and fever and scarring of the colon leading to stricture formation. Patients may become infected carriers and excrete cysts in their stools. Not all will have suffered an acute attack of dysentery. The diagnosis is made on identification of amoebae or cysts in pus or stool.

Treatment

Treatment is by metronidazole (Flagyl) in a dosage of 800 mg three times daily for 5 days. In severely ill adults and in young children it is wise to add a course of tetracycline to combat secondary infection.

An amoebic liver abscess is also treated by metronidazole, with needle aspiration if it is large.

Schistosomiasis

Schistosomiasis affects millions of people throughout the world, and is endemic in Africa, the Middle East, the Far East and Central and South America. Three species commonly produce intestinal disease: *Schistosoma mansoni, S. intercalatum* and *S. japonicum. S. mansoni* and *S. intercalatum* are found in the Middle East and Africa and *S. japonicum* in the Far East.

The life cycle involves an intermediate host, the freshwater snail. The cercariae develop in the snail and are released into fresh water where they infect man by penetration of the skin. They then enter the portal system to develop into adult worms. After sexual reproduction the female lays ova that are released into the bowel lumen or into the general circulation to reach the lung, brain, spinal cord and urinary tract. Ova excreted in the faeces develop into larvae which, provided they find their way to fresh water, then infect the intermediate host.

Clinical Features

Initially infection produces a systemic disorder. There is a short-lived skin rash on penetration by the cercariae, and after 4 weeks a general allergic reaction takes place with fever, malaise and muscle pain. Some months later the patient develops bloody diarrhoea in exacerbations and remissions. Involvement of portal venous radicles may give rise to portal hypertension (tropical splenome-galy) and pulmonary hypertension, and spinal cord disease also occurs through microvascular invasion.

The colon becomes thickened and fibrosed showing a granulomatous reaction associated with ulceration and polyp formation. Portal hypertension causes ascites, splenomegaly and oesophageal varices.

The diagnosis is made by identifying the ova in the stool or in a biopsy of the large bowel; each species can be recognised by its characteristic ova. Complement fixation and intradermal tests are less reliable methods of diagnosis. Treatment is by praziquantel (Biltricide).

Campylobacter enterocolitis

Infection by organisms of the genus *Campylobacter* has only recently been recognised as a cause of enterocolitis and there are now several reports of epidemics due to infected food, particularly certain meats and milk. In northern Europe *Campylobacter* is probably the most common cause of infective diarr-hoea, particularly among young adults and schoolchildren. It is transmitted from infected meat and milk and dogs, but human contagion is uncommon. The organism invades the mucosa of both small and large bowel and may produce endotoxins, some of which are also found in infection by *Vibrio cholerae.*

A prodromal malaise occurs in most patients after an incubation period of up to 5 days. Diarrhoea follows shortly after with the passage of watery stool and some blood. Abdominal pain is common and acute appendicitis occasionally occurs. The disease is usually self-limiting after a week or so. The sigmoidoscopic appearances are indistinguishable from ulcerative colitis.

The diagnosis is made on isolation of the organism from the stool. Treatment is usually unnecessary but if the illness lasts for a week or more erythromycin should be given. Precautions should be taken if the patient's work involves handling food.

Pseudomembranous Colitis

Antibiotic-induced diarrhoea has been recognised for many years, and in its severest form may lead to epithelial necrosis with the formation of a 'membrane' visible on sigmoidoscopy. The clinical picture varies from a mild diarrhoea to a severe form with colonic dilatation and systemic upset.

Suppression of the normal gut flora by antibiotics may lead to colonisation by pathogens, and the disease is due to the toxin produced by *Clostridium difficile,* which cannot survive competition from other organisms. Antibiotics that have

been implicated include clindamycin, lincomycin and ampicil... . Treatment is
with metronidazole or vancomycin.

Other Infections

Other infections involving the large bowel include that due to *Yersinia enterocolitis*, non-schistosomal worm infections, actinomycosis, giardiasis and tuberculosis. Infection with *Yersinia* is responsible for some cases of terminal ileitis, which
is a self-limiting condition. A summary of roundworm (nematodes) and tapeworm (cestodes) infections is given in Table 9.8. A full account is given in
textbooks on infectious and tropical diseases. Sexually transmitted diseases are
described in Chapter 5.

Radiation Enterocolitis

Radiotherapy in total doses of 40 Gy or more may cause damage to the intestine.
Its effect varies according to the energy emission, the fractionation regime and
the field irradiated. Normal tissue tolerance is greater if multiple small fractions
are given since recovery of the rapidly dividing gut epithelium is allowed. With
external beam therapy, higher-energy irradiation allows the dose to be concentrated more accurately into the volume of tissue to be treated. As far as the field
is concerned, damage to small bowel, for example, will be considerably greater
after radiotherapy to an abdominal rather than a pelvic lesion.

   Abdominal or pelvic radiotherapy has been used for uterine and bladder
cancer for some years. More recently it has been given to an increasing number of
patients with rectal cancer and there is clear evidence that, particularly after
postoperative treatment, radiation enteritis is an important hazard. This is
especially so if a loop of small bowel becomes fixed by adhesions in the field to be
treated.

Pathology

Irradiation produces an acute inflammatory response which occurs within a few
days and settles over the subsequent weeks. In some cases a chronic reaction may
be produced which becomes manifest after an interval ranging from months to
years. This may take the form of mucosal inflammation, intramural fibrosis or
necrosis.

Table 9.8. Roundworm and tapeworm infestations

Organism	Adult size (mm)	Intermediate host	Intestinal site in man	Other organ involvement	Symptoms	Diagnosis	Treatment
Nematodes							
Ascaris	100(+)	–	Large and small intestine	Lung; liver	Intestinal obstruction; cough during pulmonary migration; jaundice	Ova in stool	Piperazine
Enterobius (threadworm)	20	–	Large intestine; terminal ileum	None	Pruritus ani	Ova in stool or on skin	Piperazine
Trichuris (whipworm)	25(+)	–	Large intestine	None	Usually none	Ova in stool	Mebendazole
Strongyloides	2–3	–	Duodenum; small intestine	Lung; skin	Anorexia, weight loss, diarrhoea	Larvae in stool or duodenal aspiration	Thiabendazole, mebendazole, bephenium
Ancylostoma, Necator (hookworm)		–	Small intestine	Lung	Anaemia	Ova in stool	Mebendazole
Cestodes		*Obligatory*					
Taenia solium	2000	Pig	Small and large intestine	Muscle; brain (cysticercosis)	Usually none; nutritional deficiency	Ova and segments in stool	Niclosamide
Taenia saginata	6000	Cattle	Small and large intestine	None	Usually none; nutritional deficiency	Ova and segments in stool	Niclosamide
Diphyllobothrium latum	9000	Fish	Small and large intestine	Muscle; cysts	Vitamin B12 deficiency	Ova and segments in stool	Praziquantel
Echinococcus		Sheep→dog	Small and large intestine	Liver; lungs; pancreas; spleen	Masses due to cysts	Hydatid complement fixation test	Mebendazole ± surgery

Small Bowel

When mucosal damage predominates, radiation enteritis may cause diarrhoea and malabsorption. Fibrosis leads to stricture and adhesion formation producing obstruction.

The diagnosis is made from the history and the demonstration of abnormalities on a small bowel barium meal examination. Changes may be difficult to distinguish from features which might indicate recurrent carcinoma, and further investigation may be necessary. There may be concurrent large bowel radiation damage.

Diarrhoea is often difficult to treat satisfactorily and, if due to a diffusely involved segment of intestine, it should be managed symptomatically by anti-diarrhoeal agents. A low-fat diet may help. In cases of obstruction, laparotomy with resection of strictures or division of adhesions is indicated unless obstructive episodes settle spontaneously or are tolerably infrequent. In the latter circumstance the patient is advised to avoid certain foods, for example skins, pith and other roughage likely to provoke bolus obstruction. Resection and anastomosis of irradiated bowel is hazardous owing to its relatively poor blood supply and healing properties.

Large Bowel

The rectum and rectosigmoid are the segments of large bowel most commonly affected since they lie within the field used to treat cancer of the uterus, bladder and rectum itself. As with small bowel disease there are three broad types of presentation.

Radiation Proctitis

Mucosal damage and fibrosis of the rectal wall lead to diarrhoea, often with the passage of blood which may be severe. The sigmoidoscopic appearances include diffuse erythema, contact bleeding and ulceration, and biopsy shows non-specific inflammation. Radiation proctitis does not respond to anti-inflammatory agents or to defunctioning by a proximal colostomy. If bleeding is severe, rectal excision or some form of pull-through procedure is indicated.

Obstruction

Fibrosis causing stricture formation results in obstruction which is usually chronic and incomplete. A radiation stricture is diagnosed by endoscopy and contrast radiology after excluding malignancy and other causes of narrowing. Symptoms may be relieved by laxatives but surgical treatment is often needed. In a few cases dilatation is feasible but resection is required if symptoms persist.

Fistulation

Necrosis of the bowel wall may result in fistulation into neighbouring organs. It occurs where the absorbed dose has been particularly high and most usually affects the rectum adjacent to the vagina after intracavity irradiation of a cervical carcinoma. The resulting rectovaginal fistula causes faecal incontinence. A recto-vesical fistula may occur in males after irradiation of bladder carcinoma. A rectovaginal or rectovesical fistula can be felt on digital examination and defined radiologically. Direct closure will fail and the only prospect of cure, if a permanent colostomy is to be avoided, is by a pull-through operation bringing healthy proximal colon down to the rectum or anal canal below the level of the fistula.

A more detailed account of operations for radiation proctocolitis is given in standard textbooks.

Further Reading

Allan RN (1983) Extra-intestinal manifestations of inflammatory bowel disease. Clin Gastroenterol 12: 617–632

Allan RJ, Keighley MRB, Alexander-Williams H, Hawkins CF (eds) (1983) Inflammatory bowel diseases. Churchill Livingstone, Edinburgh

Baker WNW, Glass RE, Ritchie JK, Aylett SO (1978) Cancer of the rectum following colectomy and ileorectal anastomosis for ulcerative colitis. Br J Surg 65: 862–868

Ball AP (1982) Notes on infectious diseases. Churchill Livingstone, Edinburgh

DeCosse JJ, Rhodes RS, Wentz WB (1969) The natural history and management of radiation-induced injury of the gastrointestinal tract. Ann Surg 170: 369–384

Hodgson HJF (1980) Immunological aspects of inflammatory bowel disease. In: Brooke PV and Wilkinson A (eds) Inflammatory disease of the bowel. Pitman Medical, London, pp 38–52

Kirsner JB (1982a) Recent developments in 'nonspecific' inflammatory bowel disease: I. N Engl J Med 306: 775–785

Kirsner JB (1982b) Recent developments in 'nonspecific' inflammatory bowel disease: II. N Engl J Med 306: 837–848

Langman MJS (1979) The epidemiology of chronic intestinal disease. Edward Arnold, London

Lennard-Jones JE (1983) Toward optimal use of corticosteroids in ulcerative colitis and Crohn's disease. Gut 24: 177–181

Lennard-Jones JE, Powell-Tuck J (1979) Drug treatment of inflammatory bowel disease. Clin Gastroenterol 8: 187–217

Lennard-Jones JE, Morson BC, Ritchie JK, Shove DC, Williams CB (1977) Cancer in colitis: Assessment of the individual risk by clinical and histological criteria. Gastroenterology 73: 1280–1289

McDermott F, Hughes ESR, Pihl E (1980) Mortality and morbidity of Crohn's disease and ulcerative colitis in Australia. Med J Aust I: 534–536

Ritchie JK, Powell-Tuck J, Lennard-Jones JE (1978) Clinical outcome of the first ten years of ulcerative colitis and proctitis. Lancet I: 1140–1143

Russell JC, Welch JP (1979) Operative management of radiation injuries of the intestinal tract. Am J Surg 137: 433

Sales DJ (1983) The prognosis of inflammatory bowel disease. Arch Intern Med 143: 294–299

Shorter RG (1983) Risks of intestinal cancer in Crohn's disease. Dis Colon Rectum 26: 686–689

Skirrow MB (1977) *Campylobacter enteritis*, a new disease. Br Med J II: 9–11

Summers RW, Switz DM, Sessions JT, Becktel JM, Best WR, Kern F, Singleton JW (1979) National co-operative Crohn's disease study: Results of drug treatment. Gastroenterology 77: 847–869

Swan RW, Fowler WC, Boronow RC (1976) Surgical management of radiation injury to the small intestine. Surg Gynecol Obstet 142: 325

Tedesco FH (1980) Differential diagnosis of ulcerative colitis and Crohn's ileo-colitis and other specific inflammatory disease of the bowel. Med Clin N Am 64: 1173–1183

10 Disorders of Bowel Function

Diverticular Disease

Diverticular disease is the commonest organic colonic condition encountered. It is rare below the age of 30 but increases in incidence thereafter with one-third of patients over the age of 60 having diverticula on barium enema examination. In patients under 50 it is commoner in males and this small group is more likely to have symptoms and to develop complications, with about 50% requiring surgery. In old people it is commoner in females and surgery is needed only rarely.

Classification

Most patients with diverticula are asymptomatic and are only identified by barium enema examination. Others have symptoms and can be divided into those with uncomplicated and those with complicated diverticular disease. This last group is a minority; the possible reasons for complicated disease are given in Table 10.1. Most cases are the result of inflammation around diverticula leading to acute diverticulitis, perforation, abscess and fistula formation or stenosis. Haemorrhage is uncommon but is a major cause of massive colonic bleeding. The sigmoid colon is affected in over 90% of cases and in 65% it is the only site of disease. Diverticula do not occur in the rectum.

Table 10.1. Diverticular disease: Classification

Asymptomatic
Symptomatic
Uncomplicated
Complicated
   Acute diverticulitis
   Perforation
     Local abscess
     General peritonitis
   Fistula
   Stenosis
   Haemorrhage

Aetiology

There is evidence that diverticula develop as the result of disordered motility of the bowel. Short lengths of colon are thought to become isolated between points of segmental contraction, causing abnormally high pressures to be exerted on the bowel wall. As a consequence the mucosa herniates through the muscle at its weakest points namely the sites of entry of the blood vessels. Tensile strength of the bowel musculature diminishes with age.

In support of this theory raised sigmoid colonic intraluminal pressure has been demonstrated in patients with diverticular disease during stimulation of the colon by opiates, although under basal conditions intraluminal pressure is the same as in control subjects. A prediverticular state is said to be recognised on barium enema examination where the lumen is narrowed and the smooth haustral pattern replaced by a saw-toothed concertina-like appearance considered to be due to hypertrophy of the circular and longitudinal muscle of the bowel.

There is an epidemiological association between the prevalence of diverticular disease and the fibre content of the diet. Comparison of groups of African and English subjects has shown lower daily stool weight and longer intestinal transit in the latter. It has been suggested that this is due to low dietary fibre which results in increased sigmoid colonic activity, leading to hypertrophy of smooth muscle and raised intraluminal pressure. When individuals with and without diverticular disease in the same society are compared, however, these differences are less apparent and such studies can be criticised for not taking account of the variation in stool weight and intestinal transit times observed in the same individual from day to day.

Some workers have attempted to compare motility on the basis of an index derived from measurements of colonic activity at rest, during stimulation with prostigmine or morphine, and after food. Reports have varied from no difference to an increased motility index in patients with symptomatic diverticular disease. Bile salts stimulate colonic motility and some workers have reported higher daily output in patients with diverticular disease compared with controls.

Asymptomatic Diverticular Disease

On X-ray films diverticula may distort the bowel and obscure a neoplasm, but provided the clinician is confident that no other lesion exists, no further action is necessary. Flexible endoscopy is indicated if there is any doubt. There is no harm in recommending a high-fibre diet although any value in preventing symptoms is non-proven.

Symptomatic Diverticular Disease

Uncomplicated

DIAGNOSIS. The patient may complain of a variety of symptoms including abdominal pain, distension, constipation or diarrhoea. Some notice mucus in the stool but the passage of small amounts of blood is atypical and more suggestive of a neoplasm. The pain is usually lower abdominal and tends to be more on the left side. It may be worse after food and relieved by defaecation or the passage of flatus, and is usually dull and of several hours' duration.

Often there is tenderness over the sigmoid colon which may be palpable. Rectal digital examination may be painful and a mass may be felt.

Crohn's disease as well as carcinoma can be present in patients with diverticular disease. Anal and rectal lesions should be looked for and besides a barium enema, a barium follow-through examination and colonoscopy should be requested if the diagnosis is still suspected.

MANAGEMENT. The main diagnostic difficulty is whether the symptoms are actually ascribable to diverticular disease. Twenty years ago surgical resection for symptoms was common but the results were poor. About 20% of patients were helped but pain persisted in the majority. In many cases symptoms were in all likelihood a manifestation of the irritable bowel syndrome. There is no way at present of making this distinction other than on purely clinical grounds.

A high-fibre diet helps symptoms in many patients and early uncontrolled trials reported improvement in over 70% of cases. Fibre causes a reduction in bowel motility and intestinal transit time, making it a logical treatment on the basis of the proposed pathogenetic mechanism of high intraluminal pressure and high motility index. More recent controlled studies have shown, however, that many patients taking a placebo preparation also experience symptomatic improvement and it is therefore difficult to determine the precise value of fibre. Bran is a rich seems to be more effective than fine or cooked bran. Cereals such as All-Bran have a relatively low fibre content and crude miller's bran which is obtainable at have a relatively low fibre content and crude miller's bran which is obtainable at health shops is recommended. Two tablespoons daily sprinkled on cereal or mixed with milk are a reasonable dose. Symptoms are also helped by sterculia and ispaghula. Surgical resection is indicated when severe symptoms are not relieved and no cause other than diverticular disease can be found.

Complicated

ACUTE DIVERTICULITIS. The patient with acute diverticulitis presents with pain in the lower abdomen, malaise, anorexia and fever of a few hours to days in duration. Constipation is very common and dysuria may also occur. There are signs of local peritonitis usually in the left iliac fossa, often with a tender mass. On rectal examination a tender mass anterior to the rectum may be felt and fluctuation indicates abscess formation. The plain abdominal X-ray film is likely to show faecal loading of the colon and a soft tissue shadow with displacement of the sigmoid may also be seen. The white cell count is raised.

The differential diagnosis includes any condition causing an acute abdomen; these include gynaecological diseases and a vaginal examination should never be omitted. The patient requires admission to hospital and treatment with antibiotics. If an abscess develops it should be drained.

PERFORATION. A perforation that is contained locally will present as an abscess (see above). One that has free access to the peritoneal cavity will cause generalised peritonitis. Admission to hospital, resuscitation and urgent laparotomy are required.

FISTULA. A fistula may follow an episode of acute diverticulitis with the formation of an abscess which has become adherent to a neighbouring structure, but it may be unheralded by any previous illness. The bladder is most commonly involved but fistulas to the uterus, vagina, small bowel and skin can all occur. A colovesical fistula causes recurrent urinary infections and pneumaturia. Sometimes pieces of faecal material are passed per urethram. The symptom of pneumaturia confirms the diagnosis whether or not there is radiological evidence of a fistula. Cystoscopy may show an area of mucosal redness, usually at the dome of the bladder, but a fistulous opening is often not seen. Barium enema examination and an intravenous urogram should be carried out in all cases. An enterocutaneous fistula can be defined by sinography. The treatment is by surgical resection of the diseased bowel and fistula track.

STENOSIS. Large bowel obstruction due to diverticular disease is rare and its presence should raise suspicions of a coexisting carcinoma. Small bowel obstruction due to the adhesion of a loop of small bowel to an area of diverticular disease is more common.

BLEEDING. Bleeding is uncommon in diverticular disease. It is usually major and may cause shock. The diagnosis should be suspected when large volumes of unchanged blood and fresh clots are passed. Patients with bleeding often have diverticula of both right and left colon and it has been suggested that right-sided diverticula may be associated with angiodysplasia in this site.

Other lesions causing major haemorrhage include carcinoma, inflammatory bowel disease and haemorrhoids. The patient should be admitted to hospital and bleeding from the upper gastrointestinal tract excluded by gastroscopy. In an actively bleeding patient, selective angiography may identify the site. Bleeding usually settles spontaneously, but if it does not, laparotomy should be undertaken. A total colectomy should be performed since bleeding may be coming from either the right or left colon, usually the former.

The Irritable Bowel Syndrome

The irritable bowel syndrome is the commonest disorder with no known organic cause presenting to gastroenterologists. It is a distinct clinical entity which includes a complex of symptoms but no abnormality on examination or investigation. Although a benign condition, the symptoms may severely disturb the patient's life. Alternative terms include functional bowel disease, irritable colon, spastic colon and mucous colitis, but the disorder is not confined to the colon and patients may present with symptoms referable to any part of the gastrointestinal tract.

Aetiology

Although the aetiology is unknown, patients often show anxiety, tension or aggression and may be depressed. Some date the onset to an attack of 'food poisoning' or acute diarrhoea and 15% will admit to purgative abuse suggesting a long-standing disorder. Increased motor activity in the colon in response to emotional stimulation or the administration of drugs that stimulate the bowel has been demonstrated and symptoms in some patients improve with antispasmodic agents. Many consider that the condition represents an exaggeration of normal function with disordered and unco-ordinated colonic activity. It is interesting that the reaction of the normal bowel to experimentally induced stress includes a marked increase in motility, hyperaemia and an excess production of mucus. Present research into hormonal, motility and biochemical variables in patients with the irritable bowel syndrome may increase our understanding of the disorder.

Diagnosis

Symptoms

Females are affected twice as frequently as males, and some have had a previous abdominal operation such as a gynaecological procedure or appendicectomy.

The patient complains of a combination of abdominal pain, abdominal distension, diarrhoea or constipation. Abdominal pain is experienced by most patients at some time. It can occur in any part of the abdomen but most commonly in the left flank and the left iliac fossa. Pain may occur outside the abdomen, for example in the chest, back and buttocks, and can be produced by colonic distension caused by insufflation of air during colonoscopy. The pain may be aggravated by food and some subjects seem to have a particular food intolerance. Night pain is, however, rare. Abdominal distension, constipation with the passage of small hard dry pellet stools, or diarrhoea sometimes with explosive defaecation may occur. Occasionally mucus alone is passed after defaecation.

Some patients complain of indigestion and epigastric fullness after meals. The symptoms of the irritable bowel syndrome can also be produced by serious disease. Particular features suggesting organic conditions include the onset of symptoms over the age of 40, progression of symptoms, occurrence of symptoms at night, and weight loss or bleeding.

Examination and Investigation

There may be abdominal distension and tenderness usually in the right iliac fossa. Anorectal examination is normal. Although the barium enema examination sometimes shows prominent haustral markings associated with areas of segmental spasm no localised lesion can be demonstrated. The administration of intravenous antispasmodics during the examination usually relaxes the bowel and allows filling of contracted segments. Small bowel barium meal, cholecystography and excretion urography may be necessary to exclude disease in these organs.

Treatment

The most useful aspect of treatment is to be able to reassure the patient that there is no serious disease such as cancer. Since the cause is unknown it is difficult to advise specific treatment. It may help some patients to appreciate that their symptoms are the result of an exaggerated but normal response to stress. Antispasmodic drugs, sedatives, peppermint oil preparations and antidepressants may relieve pain and distension. Constipation should be treated by hydrophilic bulking agents but irritant laxatives should be avoided. Codeine phosphate or loperamide will relieve diarrhoea in some patients.

The overall results of treatment are disappointing since only one-third of patients gain relief of symptoms.

Slow Transit Constipation

A group of patients has been recognised with severe constipation, a normal barium enema examination, an intact anorectal reflex and a reduction in intestinal transit time. The condition occurs almost exclusively in females, who usually present in early adult life. The pathogenesis is unknown but there may be abnormalities of colonic smooth muscle function, and in some patients amenorrhoea with abnormal sex hormone levels has been described.

Most patients can be treated by diet or laxatives. If medical treatment fails surgery may help; colectomy with ileorectal anastomosis is the operation of choice, with about 50% of patients gaining long-lasting relief of symptoms.

Normal Transit Constipation

Most patients with constipation will have a normal anorectal reflex, normal barium enema examination and a normal wholegut transit time. The condition probably represents a variant of the irritable bowel syndrome, with difficulty in evacuation as the chief symptom. Straining with the frequent passage of small rabbit-like stools or intermittent episodes of explosive diarrhoea are often present. Some patients develop weakness of the pelvic floor possibly secondary to chronic straining.

Management should be medical by dietary changes and bulk laxatives such as bran, ispaghula and sterculia. If abdominal symptoms are present, sedatives and antispasmodics may help.

Megacolon

Aganglionic Megacolon

There are two forms of aganglionic megacolon. Hirschsprung's disease is due to a congenital absence of ganglia in the myenteric plexus of the bowel and Chagas' disease is acquired through destruction of the same ganglia by the parasite *Trypanosoma cruzi.*

Hirschsprung's Disease

Most cases of Hirschsprung's disease present in infancy but occasionally the patient will not seek medical help until adolescence or adulthood. Males suffer nine times more often than females and a sibling is affected in about 10% of cases. There is an association between Hirschsprung's disease and Down's syndrome.

PATHOLOGY. There are two histological abnormalities. First, ganglia are absent from the myenteric plexus of the affected bowel, and secondly there is an increase in the numbers of non-myelinated nerve fibres in the submucosa. The most distal part of the rectum is always affected and the lesion extends proximally over a variable distance. In 10% of cases the rectum only is involved and in 95% the disease does not extend beyond the proximal sigmoid colon. Total colonic and rectal disease is rare. Occasionally only a few centimetres of distal rectum are involved (ultrashort segment).

At the proximal end of the affected segment ganglia begin to be seen. The numbers increase gradually over a distance of a few centimetres until normal bowel is reached. The affected bowel is in a state of spasm and is referred to as the spastic segment. As a result, there is a functional obstruction to the passage of faeces and the normal proximal bowel distends.

DIAGNOSIS. Constipation occurs in all cases, the severity depending to some degree on the length of the spastic segment. The abdomen is distended and faecal loading is readily palpable. Distension may be so great that the ribs become splayed and respiration embarrassed. Faecal soiling does not occur. In infancy the picture is usually of intestinal obstruction with weight loss and anorexia. In older individuals constipation may not be so severe, but even in adults it can almost always be traced back to early childhood.

The anal sphincter feels tight in one-third of patients and the rectum is often collapsed seeming to grip the examining finger. Sigmoidoscopy often reveals a collapsed rectum and it may be possible to enter dilated bowel above the spastic segment.

INVESTIGATION. The differential diagnosis lies between other forms of megacolon (Table 10.2) and diseases which cause constipation.

A plain X-ray film of the abdomen will show gross distension with faecal loading of the colon, most usually as far as the sigmoid—unlike the situation in diverticular disease, irritable bowel syndrome and medical diseases such as myxoedema. A barium enema examination will demonstrate dilation above the narrowed distal segment. The lateral view of the rectum is an important part of this examination since the transitional zone (cone) between the spastic and dilated bowel is often best demonstrated in this way. In adults this area should be examined carefully for signs of a carcinoma.

The rectosphincteric inhibition reflex does not occur in Hirschsprung's disease, which is the only form of constipation or megacolon showing this feature. The test is more sensitive than any other in making the diagnosis (Fig. 3.3, p.45). However, histological confirmation of the diagnosis is also necessary. In infants a mucosal biopsy is sufficient but in adults the pathologist needs a full thickness sample under a general anaesthetic, taking the biopsy at a point just above the anorectal junction. A false positive result may occur if the biopsy is taken from the anal canal where ganglia are normally not found.

MANAGEMENT. The treatment is surgical, and the reader is referred to surgical textbooks. The various operations all attempt to remove as much of the aganglionic segment as is possible whilst retaining pelvic floor function, bringing

Table 10.2. Differential diagnosis of Hirschsprung's disease and idiopathic megacolon

	Hirschsprung's disease	Idiopathic megacolon
Clinical assessment		
Duration of constipation	Usually from infancy	Usually from childhood or later
Soiling	Never	Frequent
Anal sphincter	Tonic	Lax
Rectum	Collapsed	Ballooned
Investigation		
Barium enema	Spastic segment ± cone	Ballooned rectum
Rectosphincteric reflex	Absent	Present
Histology	Cholinergic nerve fibres increased; absent or a few ganglia	Normal

proximal normal bowel down to the level of the anorectal junction. The rare cases of ultrashort segment Hirschsprung's disease can be treated by an extended internal sphincterotomy. Acute cases, which are unlikely to present to the rectal clinic, all occur in infants and require specialist paediatric care.

Chagas' Disease

Chagas' disease is common in Brazil and is caused by the protozoon *Trypanosoma cruzi*. The organism is present in the reservoir hosts of dog, cat or armadillo and is transmitted to man through bites of the infected vector, the triatomol fly.

Ganglionic degeneration, probably caused by a toxin, takes place throughout the body. The effect is greatest in the myocardium, oesophagus and distal large bowel, producing a cardiomyopathy, abnormal oesophageal motility and megacolon and megarectum. Constipation and abdominal distension are progressive. There is no specific cure and patients may require colonic resection for constipation.

Idiopathic Megacolon

Investigation of constipation will identify a group of subjects with dilatation of the colon or rectum or both without apparent cause or histological abnormality. Cases can be divided into those with a dilated rectum and those with a dilated colon but normal rectum.

Megarectum

Megarectum usually presents in childhood and probably develops through neglecting the call to stool with resulting rectal distension and loss of rectal sensation. Fear of defaecation may play some part especially if a painful anal lesion such as a fissure is present. There is no increased familial incidence and no sex difference when the condition presents in childhood, but in adult life the condition occurs more often in males. About 20% of patients are mentally deficient or suffer from a personality disorder and there is often a family history of unhappiness or psychological tension. Soiling is a frequent feature, in contrast to Hirschsprung's disease.

The anus is usually lax and the rectum impacted and capacious. There are no histological abnormalities and the myenteric ganglia are normal. A plain abdominal X-ray film often shows gross faecal loading in the rectum and distal colon, and megarectum can be confirmed by a barium contrast enema examination. Anorectal physiology shows a normal rectosphincteric reflex.

Management

Megarectum is difficult to treat but the chance of success is greater if the history is short. The bowel should be emptied by enemas and washouts and manual disimpaction may be necessary. The aim is then to initiate a regular pattern of defaecation, which will require an appreciation by the patient or patient's parents of the problem and the regular use of a laxative such as magnesium sulphate (Epsom salts). Glycerine or bisacodyl (Dulcolax) suppositories or a phosphate enema to keep the rectum empty can also be prescribed. Surgery gives poor results and the treatment of any psychological factors is most important.

Megacolon

Idiopathic megacolon is uncommon, and mostly affects females. It presents later in life than megarectum, usually between 20 and 50 years of age, and the cause is unknown. Barium enema examination shows dilatation of all or part of the colon.

Management

Patients should be treated with regular aperients such as magnesium sulphate or bisacodyl and some cases are improved by suppositories or disposable enemas in addition. Surgical treatment should be avoided unless medical treatment has failed, when a few patients are helped by colectomy and ileorectal anastomosis.

Further Reading

Abrahamsson H (1982) Irritable bowel syndrome: Diagnosis. Scand J Gastroenterol [Suppl] 79: 20–23
Bentley SJ (1983) Food hypersensitivity in irritable bowel syndrome. Lancet II: 295–297
Burkitt DP, Trowill HC (1975) Refined carbohydrate foods and disease. Academic Press, London
Dotevill G (1982) Treatment of irritable bowel syndrome. Scand J Gastroenterol [Suppl] 79: 124–127
Eastwood MA, Watters DAK, Smith AN (1982) Diverticular disease: Is it a motility disorder? Clin Gastroenterol 11: 545–561
Gledhill T, Hunt RH (1983) Bleeding and diverticular disease. Lancet I: 830
Heaton KW (1984) Irritable bowel syndrome. In: Bouchier IAD, Allan RN, Hodgson HJF, Keighley MRB (eds) Textbook of gastroenterology. Baillière Tindall, London, pp 867–875
Hinton JM, Lennard-Jones JE, Young AC (1969) A new method for studying gut transit times using radioopaque markers. Gut 10: 842–847
Lawson JON (1984) Hirschsprung's disease. In: Bouchier IAD, Allan RN, Hodgson HJF, Keighley MRB (eds) Textbook of gastroenterology. Baillière Tindall, London, pp 751–765
Martelli H, Devroide G, Arhan P, Dugnay C, Dornic C, Faverdin C (1978) Some parameters of large bowel motility in normal man. Gastroenterology 75: 612–618
Murney RG, Winship DH (1982) The irritable colon syndrome. Clin Gastroenterol 11: 563–592
Olness K, McParland FA, Piper J (1980) Biofeedback: A new modality in the management of children with fecal soiling. J Pediat 96: 505–509
Painter NS, Truelove SC (1964) The intraluminal pressure patterns in diverticulosis of the colon. Gut 5: 201–213
Parks TG (1969) Natural history of diverticular disease of the colon. A review of 521 cases. Br Med J IV: 639–642

Preston DM, Hawley PR, Lennard-Jones JE, Todd IP (1984) Results of colectomy for severe idiopathic constipation in women (Arbuthnot Lane's disease). Br J Surg 71: 547–552
Svedlund J (1983) Controlled study of psychotherapy in irritable bowel syndrome. Lancet II: 589–592
Swarbrick ET, Hegarty JE, Bat L, Williams CB (1980) Site of pain from the irritable bowel. Lancet II: 443–446
Thompson WG (1984) The irritable bowel. Gut 25: 305–320
Weinreich J (1982) Treatment of diverticular disease. Scand J Gastroenterol [Suppl] 79: 128–129
Whitehead WE, Schuster MM (1981) Behavioural approaches to the treatment of gastrointestinal motility disorders. Med Clin N Am 65: 1397–1411

11 Vascular Disorders

Malformations

With the development of selective angiography and flexible endoscopy vascular malformations are now recognised to be an important cause of large bowel haemorrhage. Their prevalence is not known since the diagnosis is made only after investigation of bleeding. It seems reasonable at the present time to divide them into congenital and acquired malformations. The former are rare, while the latter, generally known as angiodysplasia, appear to be fairly common.

Congenital Malformations

Some haemangiomas are congenital. There may be a long history of persistent anaemia going back to childhood, with a positive family history in a few patients. Intestinal vascular malformations may occasionally be accompanied by oral and cutaneous lesions (hereditary telangiectasia, Osler-Rendu disease) or very rarely by similar lesions in the limbs (Weber-Klippel disease).

Patients present either with anaemia due to chronic blood loss or with massive haemorrhage. Any part of the gastrointestinal tract may be affected, the small bowel most commonly (50%), followed by stomach (40%) and large bowel (25%). The lesions may be single or multiple and vary from the size of a pin-head to several centimetres, sometimes affecting a long segment of intestine. The full thickness of the bowel may be involved, but those lesions causing bleeding lie within the submucosa and mucosa. The lesion may extend into surrounding fat and neighbouring organs. Calcification, usually due to phlebolith formation, may occur.

The diagnosis is made either on endoscopy or by selective angiography. Contrast barium examinations are of no value. Cavernous haemangiomas of the rectum can be seen on sigmoidoscopy as dilated tortuous veins in the submucosa.

Acquired Malformations

Angiodysplasia

Angiodysplasia was recognised only after the introduction of selective angiography. The lesions are not visible on macroscopic examination of resected specimens but can be demonstrated on histological examination after injection of the specimen with silicone rubber and barium paste compounds. They are usually only a few millimetres in size and consist of dilated submucosal vascular spaces. Mucosal involvement may occur and arteriovenous shunts have been described. The lesions almost always appear to be in the caecum and ascending colon.

Angiodysplasia is thought to be an acquired condition possibly due to degeneration of blood vessel walls. The disease is usually seen in old people, although young adults may be affected. It has been suggested that venous congestion due to increased intramural muscle tension may lead to dilatation of submucosal veins, and it may be that the association between right-sided diverticular disease and bleeding is due to coexisting angiodysplasia.

DIAGNOSIS. Patients often give a history of previous investigation for gastrointestinal bleeding and a previous abdominal operation such as gastrectomy or partial colectomy is not uncommon.

When bleeding is minor and intermittent the diagnosis should be considered in any patient with a normal barium enema examination. Colonoscopy is indicated and although a colonic neoplasm will be the commonest lesion discovered, about 30%–50% of such patients will be found to have angiodysplasia. A small area of tortuous dilated submucosal vessels or of non-ulcerated reddening is seen.

Persistent bleeding with a normal colonoscopy is an indication for gastroscopy and small bowel contrast radiology. If these are normal, selective angiography should be carried out. This may demonstrate the lesion in the area of distribution of the blood vessels to the right colon.

In patients who present with major bleeding emergency colonoscopy has been advocated by some endoscopists but others have not found it helpful since vision is often obscured by blood. After gastroscopy, selective angiography is the investigation of choice and barium studies are contraindicated since residual barium will mask any features on the angiogram. The site of an actively bleeding lesion may be seen as a blush of extravasated contrast if the rate of blood loss is over about 1 ml/min. In the last few years radiolabelled red cell scintigraphy has been used to localise the site and is now the investigation of choice when bleeding is actually occurring.

TREATMENT. Treatment is by surgical resection. In the elective case right hemicolectomy will satisfactorily remove the lesion. However a total colectomy is the operation of choice in cases of acute haemorrhage which has failed to stop spontaneously, since bleeding may be due to lesions other than angiodysplasia (for example diverticular disease).

Ischaemic Bowel Disease

The proximal colon receives blood via branches of the superior mesenteric artery and the distal bowel receives its supply from branches of the inferior mesenteric artery and internal iliac arteries. Unlike the small bowel, which is supplied by a series of vascular arcades, the large bowel has a relatively poor blood supply. It relies largely on the marginal artery, particularly if there is occlusion of a major vessel. There is a 'watershed' between the supply from the superior mesenteric and the inferior mesenteric vessels at the splenic flexure and it is at this site that ischaemic damage is most often seen.

Aetiology

Table 11.1 summarises the common causes of large bowel ischaemia. The inferior mesenteric artery is frequently blocked by atheroma but a collateral blood supply usually develops. If this is interrupted or embarrassed in any way, then ischaemia may result. Ischaemia may follow surgery for aortic aneurysms but this is an unusual event as the inferior mesenteric artery is already thrombosed in the majority of patients. Small blood vessels can become occluded in patients with primary vascular disorders or after radiotherapy. The blood supply may become critical if flow is further reduced by heart failure, intravascular coagulation or intestinal obstruction. Extensive venous thrombosis has been considered to produce large bowel ischaemia and there is circumstantial evidence to incriminate oral contraceptives.

Table 11.1 Large bowel ischaemia: Causes

Occlusion of major vessels	Surgical ligation
	Atheroma
	Spontaneous thrombosis
	Embolism
	Trauma
Occlusion of small vessels	Polyarteritis
	Rheumatoid arthritis
	Connective tissue disorders
	Radiotherapy
Contributing factors	Intestinal obstruction
	Low flow states
	Intravascular coagulation

Pathology

A single segment of bowel, most commonly in the splenic flexure, sigmoid or rectosigmoid, is involved, the length ranging from a few centimetres to the entire left colon. The rectum is only rarely affected.

The severity of ischaemia depends on the degree of occlusion and its duration. Recovery of the blood supply may occur if the collateral circulation is adequate or if the cardiac output improves. The effects of ischaemia are compounded by the presence of bacteria in the lumen which accelerate necrosis. Complete unrelenting ischaemia leads to gangrene of the bowel while a transient episode produces an inflammatory picture which may undergo complete resolution or heal by repair to leave a fibrous stricture. The mucosa is the layer of the bowel most sensitive to ischaemia and in the acute non-gangrenous condition becomes oedematous and ulcerated with the formation of intramural haemorrhages. After extensive damage but where the ischaemia is not severe enough to cause gangrene, organisation and fibrosis occur, and macrophages containing large amounts of haemosiderin are a characteristic feature.

Diagnosis

Symptoms

Patients are usually elderly and frequently have cardiac problems. The effect of colonic ischaemia depends on its degree. When gangrene results, the patient presents gravely ill as an emergency. An attack of transient ischaemia presents as an acute illness of sudden onset, most usually with left-sided abdominal pain, diarrhoea and the passage of blood and mucus. The illness may last from a few days to a week and usually subsides completely. When a stricture forms, features of chronic large bowel obstruction occur after the acute condition has subsided.

Signs

There may be abdominal tenderness and rigidity localised over the affected segment, with tachycardia and pyrexia. The white cell count is frequently raised, sometimes greatly.

The involved segment is usually too proximal to be seen on rigid sigmoidoscopy, but blood, mucus and liquid stool may be present in the lumen. The rectum itself is unlikely to be affected. The lesion may, however, be seen on flexible endoscopy as an extensive area of bleeding, oedematous and ulcerated mucosa.

Investigations

A barium enema examination is indicated provided there is no evidence of perforation. The lumen is narrowed by swelling due to oedema, intramural haemorrhage and spasm and its profile is irregular, often taking the form of polypoid filling defects caused by oedematous mucosa ('thumb printing'). Spasm results not only in narrowing but also in the loss of haustral pattern and the bowel fails to distend on screening. These changes may be seen on a plain X-ray film of the abdomen with air acting as the contrast medium.

Differential Diagnosis

In the acute stage, ischaemic bowel disease may resemble an acute exacerbation of ulcerative colitis or Crohn's disease, acute diverticular disease, bowel perforation, acute pancreatitis or a leaking abdominal aneurysm. The features most helpful in making the diagnosis are: coexisting cardiovascular disease, the abrupt onset, normal rectum, absence of anal lesions and the single segment involvement shown on contrast radiology. The detailed radiological features of the affected segment are characteristic in most cases, although it may be difficult in some cases to rule out Crohn's disease.

Management

The patient should be admitted to hospital. Those with gangrene require urgent resuscitation and laparotomy as soon as possible.

Those with non-gangrenous disease should be observed for signs of deterioration and maintained on an intravenous infusion. Usually the condition settles, giving an opportunity for investigation to confirm the diagnosis. In three-quarters of the cases all clinical and radiological signs disappear. In one-quarter some degree of narrowing or deformity of the bowel persists but only occasionally is it necessary to carry out resection of a stricture.

Further Reading

Boley SJ, Sammartano R, Brandt LJ, Sprayregen S (1979) Vascular ectasias of the colon. Surg Gynecol Obstet 149: 353–359

Bookstein JJ, Noderi MJ, Walter JF (1978) Transcatheter embolisation for lower GI bleeding. Radiology 127: 345–349

Camilleri M, Chadwick VS, Hodgson HJF (1984) Vascular anomalies of the gastrointestinal tract. Hepato-gastroenterol 31: 149–153

Drapanas T, Pennington DG, Kappelman M et al. (1973) Emergency subtotal colectomy, the preferred approach to the management of massively bleeding diverticular disease. Ann Surg 177: 519–526

[Editorial] (1981) Angiodysplasia. Lancet II: 1086

Galloway SJ, Casarella WJ, Shimkin PM (1974) Vascular malformations of the right colon as a cause of bleeding in patients with aortic stenosis. Radiology 113: 11–15

Marston A (1977) Intestinal ischaemia. Edward Arnold, London

Rossini FP, Ferrari A (1981) Emergency colonoscopy. In: Hunt RH, Waye JD (eds) Colonoscopy. Chapman and Hall, London

12 Non-alimentary Pelvic Disease

It is inevitable that patients referred to a rectal clinic will sometimes be found to have non-alimentary pelvic disease and it is important in taking the history to obtain details of menstruation, abnormal vaginal bleeding and urinary symptoms.

Gynaecological Disorders

Uterine Prolapse

A number of patients with rectal prolapse or faecal incontinence will have either a rectocoele, cystocoele or complete uterine prolapse. The conditions may have a common aetiology and it is perhaps surprising that there is little common ground between gynaecologist and proctologist when considering their surgical treatment. With a better understanding of pelvic floor physiology this may be rectified.

Cystocoele

In cystocoele the anterior vaginal wall prolapses through the vulval orifice especially if the patient is asked to cough or strain. The bladder is pulled down with the vaginal prolapse leading to urinary symptoms including stress incontinence and incomplete micturition. If symptomatic, an anterior colporrhaphy should be advised.

Rectocoele

In rectocoele the posterior vaginal wall prolapses through the vulval orifice bringing the rectum with it. The sac of rectum produced may come to contain faeces, causing symptoms of incomplete defaecation and perianal discomfort. Repair is by performing a posterior colporrhaphy.

Procidentia

In procidentia the uterus prolapses between the levator muscles, turns the vagina inside out and appears at the vulval orifice. There is weakness of the transverse cervical ligaments which run between the sacrum and the cervix and lateral fornices of the vagina. The patient usually complains of 'something coming down' and occasionally may even be referred as a case of rectal prolapse. Treatment is by surgical repair often combined with hysterectomy.

Carcinoma of the Uterus

Intestinal symptoms may predominate in carcinoma of the uterus where there is extensive local invasion of the bowel, but there is usually intermenstrual or postcoital bleeding as well. Occasionally a cancer of the cervix may be found solely on anorectal examination as an anterior mass, particularly if it is invading the rectum. Tumours of the body of the uterus rarely produce symptoms other than bleeding but they sometimes invade the upper rectum, sigmoid colon or ileum, causing symptoms of stenosis or ulceration. Diagnosis requires a full gynaecological examination, cervical smear cytology and histological examination of uterine curettings.

Patients previously treated by radiotherapy for uterine carcinoma may present with proctitis, stricture or fistula formation.

Endometriosis

Endometriosis is a proliferation of functioning endometrial tissue outside the uterine cavity. The aetiology is unknown. It is limited to reproductive life, but patients are usually over 30 years of age. There is often a family history and many patients are infertile.

Endometriosis can involve the gastrointestinal tract, the urinary tract, the vault of the vagina and rarely extrapelvic metastatic sites such as the umbilicus, laparotomy scars and lymph nodes. The most common site of intestinal involvement is the rectovaginal septum, but it can occur in the lateral ligaments of the rectum or around the sigmoid colon. The lesions are usually typical chocolate cysts scattered on the serosa, but they can encircle the bowel to produce a stricture that on barium enema examination or even laparotomy may be indistinguishable from a carcinoma.

Clinical Features

The commonest symptom of endometriosis affecting the bowel is pelvic or rectal pain. This may be constant but is often aggravated by defaecation and may be related to menstruation. A mass may be palpated in the pouch of Douglas or in the rectovaginal septum. Some surgeons advocate examining the patient 24 hours before menstruation as the lesion may be more prominent and tender at this time. Laparoscopy is mandatory to confirm the diagnosis if medical treatment is to be used.

Management

Endometriosis can be treated by medical or surgical means. For many years patients have been given continuous doses of oestrogen–progesterone preparations to induce a pseudopregnancy. An alternative is to prescribe cyclic oral contraceptives with a high progesterone content. More recently a synthetic derivative of ethinyltestosterone (danazol) which produces a pseudomenopause has been used. Mild androgenic side effects may occur. Patients with bowel strictures, however, will require surgical resection. This may involve a low anterior resection if the lesion is distal.

Ovarian Masses

Like uterine carcinoma, malignant ovarian tumours may present with bowel symptoms if they have invaded the intestine. Usually they are obstructive in type. Ovarian masses are occasionally felt on digital examination per rectum and if suspected a vaginal examination must be performed. Their pathology and management are described in gynaecological textbooks.

Urological Disorders

Some bowel diseases may involve the urinary tract. Cancer of the rectum sometimes invades the bladder and prostate and fistulas into the bladder can occur from Crohn's disease, diverticular disease or cancer. Carcinoma may cause ureteric obstruction.

Patients with prostatitis sometimes present with perineal and anal pain. Urinary symptoms may be present but this is not always the case. Tenderness

over the prostate suggests the diagnosis and a midstream specimen of urine
should be sent for culture. Patients with prostatic carcinoma can present with
pelvic pain from bony secondaries. Rarely the tumour encircles the rectum and
may be mistaken for a rectal cancer, but mucosal ulceration is usually absent.
The investigation of prostatic disease is described in urological textbooks.

Presacral Tumours and Cysts

Presacral tumours are rare. They may be solid or cystic. Some cause anorectal
symptoms, some are asymptomatic and some give rise to pain, usually through
nerve compression or infiltration.

Lesions can be classified into developmental (60%), neurogenic (10%), osseous
(5%–10%) and others. The most common include:

Chordoma
Bony tumour of the sacrum or pelvis
Post-rectal dermoid
Duplication of the rectum

Any tumour of nerve or connective tissue may, however, give rise to a presacral
mass and there is a long list of pathological types.

Diagnosis

Symptoms

The symptoms depend on the size and position of the tumour and the presence or
absence of infection. Often such tumours are asymptomatic and may be
discovered by chance during examination for some other cause.

Pain is usually a feature of malignant or infected cysts. It is felt in the lower
back or as an ache in the rectum. With nerve involvement the pain may radiate
into the buttocks, hips or legs. Infection may cause fever and local pain and may
occur in repeated bouts of perianal suppuration similar to fistula-in-ano.

The tumour or cyst may be sufficiently large to interfere with the function of
other pelvic organs. Thus the rectum may be compressed and the patient
complain of constipation or incomplete evacuation, while pressure on the bladder
may cause urinary symptoms. A presacral tumour may first present during
labour.

Signs and Investigations

Digital examination per rectum will determine whether the tumour is solid or cystic and mobile or fixed. Its size and level in the pelvis should also be assessed. Sigmoidoscopy is usually unhelpful. A plain X-ray film of the pelvis will show any calcified elements and a computerised tomographic scan will define the extent. An excretion urogram is indicated if an obstructive uropathy is suspected.

Differential Diagnosis

SOLID TUMOURS. A *chordoma* is a tumour of remnants of the embryological notochord. It is commoner in males and most usually presents in late middle age. The diagnosis is made on examination of a biopsy which can be taken as a needle biopsy via the perineum or rectum. The tumour is radioresistant and treatment is by surgical excision which is best carried out by a colorectal surgeon and neurosurgeon together. There is a high rate of local recurrence.

Bony tumours are easily seen on plain X-ray films. The histological diagnosis is made by open biopsy and treatment is by radiotherapy or surgical excision depending on the size and type of tumour. A benign osteoma should, however, be treated only if it is causing symptoms.

CYSTIC TUMOURS. A *post-rectal dermoid* presents as a mobile cystic retrorectal swelling. The condition is benign and is probably a sequestration cyst originating from the time of embryological fusion of ectodermal layers. It is best removed by an abdominal approach with mobilisation of the rectum. If the cyst is small and in the lower pelvis, removal is sometimes possible through a perineal approach via the intersphincteric space.

The signs of *duplication of the rectum* are indistinguishable from those of a dermoid cyst and the diagnosis is usually made at laparotomy. Duplication may extend proximally into the colon and into the small intestine in some cases. Resection is indicated.

Appendix A. **Stomas**

Despite the increasing use of sphincter-saving operations, a stoma is unavoidable for many patients. Their quality of life has improved in the last 10–15 years, first by the introduction of disposable adhesive appliances and secondly through the services of trained stomatherapists who are available to help with practical and psychological difficulties.

The success of the stoma depends greatly on its site, which should be well away from skin creases (including the umbilicus), previous surgical wounds and bony prominences. It must be visible to the patient and easily accessible for fitting the appliances. The site should be marked preoperatively with waterproof ink with the patient standing and a disposable bag applied immediately. The patient can try sitting, bending and walking to get the feel of the appliance, and an unsatisfactory position can then be changed.

Appliances (Fig. A.1)

All appliances consist of a bag and a flange which is attached to the skin around the stoma. They are inseparable in a one-piece appliance but can be detached from each other in a two-piece appliance. Disposable bags have largely replaced non-disposable appliances. Appliances can be drainable or non-drainable and both are available as a one- or two-piece unit. A drainable appliance should be used for an ileostomy, where the stool is fluid, whereas for a sigmoid colostomy producing solid faeces a non-drainable bag is more suitable.

The two-piece appliance has the advantage that the flange is left attached to the skin while the bag is changed, and if a satisfactory seal is maintained it can be kept in place for several days. This makes management easier as it is less time-

DRAINABLE

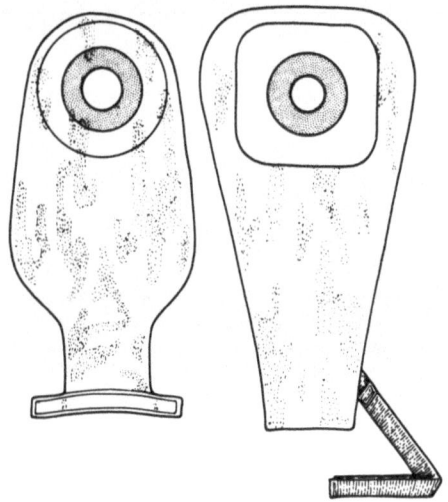
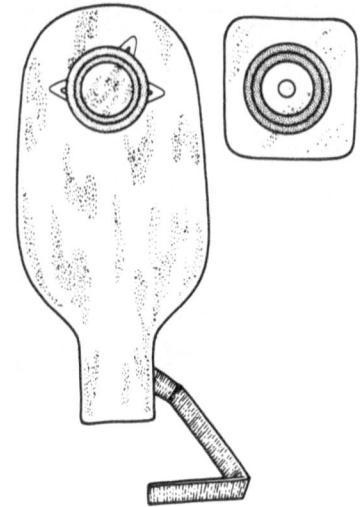

Adheres directly to skin   Separate adhesive flange
SYSTEM 1   SYSTEM 2

NON-DRAINABLE

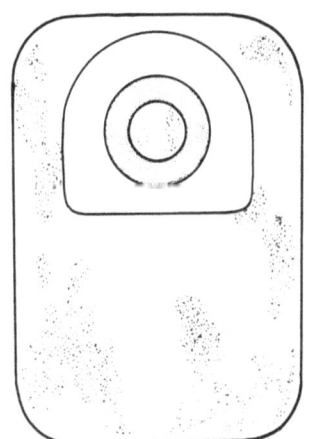

SYSTEM 1   SYSTEM 2

Fig. A.1. Basic stoma appliances.

consuming and less damaging to the skin. Most flanges have attachments for a supporting belt for added security.

Accessories

Adhesive sheeting consisting of sodium carboxymethyl cellulose, polyisobutylene, gelatin and pectin (Stomahesive) is non-reactive to skin and can stick to moist surfaces, be moulded to skin contour and easily cut with scissors. It is incorporated into the flange of some appliances but can also be obtained as separate sheets 10 cm square.

Karaya paste is useful for filling small defects between the stoma and flange, especially where there is irregularity of skin contour. Several barrier creams to protect the skin and deodorants are available. Gas which may cause bulging of the appliance or detachment of the flange can be released by puncturing the bag with a needle and covering the site with a charcoal filter; this allows flatus to escape while trapping its odoriferous elements.

Ileostomy

An ileostomy may be permanent or temporary. A permanent ileostomy results after proctocolectomy where the anal sphincter has been removed; it is therefore an end ileostomy. A temporary ileostomy is usually fashioned as a loop. Either should be constructed to form a spout about 2–3 cm long to allow the effluent to drain without contact with skin.

Complications

Skin Problems

Skin problems may arise from allergy to the appliance or from contact with small bowel effluent.

Occasionally the skin may be allergic to substances within the adhesive of the flange. Allergy should be suspected if the area of dermatitis corresponds with the area in contact with the appliance. The appliance should be removed, the skin gently cleaned and Stomahesive or a karaya sheet applied before resiting the bag. Steroid creams may be of some help. Occasionally there may be *Candida* infection of the peristomal skin.

There are several causes of leakage including a poorly fitting appliance, irregular skin contour and retraction or ulceration of the stoma. The first two are common problems which may be solved simply by changing the size of the appliance or overcoming skin irregularities with karaya paste or Stomahesive. Retraction will require refashioning, and resiting of the ileostomy may be necessary if contour difficulties are insurmountable. Ulceration at the mucocutaneous junction may cause bleeding and discharge which can lift the flange from the skin. Sometimes it is due to pressure from a flange that is too tight.

Ileostomy Dysfunction

Excessive output from the ileostomy may produce water and electrolyte (especially sodium) depletion. A persistently high output (> 1000 ml/24 hours) may be due to mechanical obstruction, non-obstructing small bowel disease, pancreatic disease, drugs or diet. Mechanical obstruction may be caused by adhesions, strictures, food bolus or stenosis of the stoma. Non-obstructing small bowel disease includes inflammation (e.g. due to Crohn's disease) and the short bowel syndrome. Common drugs producing diarrhoea include laxatives and antibiotics and alcohol in some cases. Certain foods, e.g. vegetables (especially onions) and fruits, may also do so. Often, however, no cause is found, and symptomatic treatment should be tried. Bulk laxatives thicken the stool, but increase sodium and water output. Codeine, loperamide and diphenoxylate with atropine (Lomotil) may slow transit and reduce volume.

Other Complications

Prolapse and parastomal hernia occasionally occur and should be repaired. Stenosis is fairly common and may be due to ischaemia or recurrent Crohn's disease. It may be possible to manage by dilatation but refashioning is often necessary.

Continent Ileostomy

In the continent abdominal ileostomy with ileal reservoir, the stoma is flush with the skin and emptying is achieved by catheterisation. A large-bore catheter with rounded tip and side hole is most suitable but some patients may find the bend at the tip of a bicoudé catheter easier to pass. Failure to enter the reservoir or difficulty in doing so suggests subluxation or prolapse of the nipple valve and refashioning may be necessary.

Colostomy

A colostomy may also be permanant or temporary. A permanent end colostomy results after excision of the rectum and anal canal, usually for cancer, and is formed by the sigmoid colon. A temporary loop colostomy is used to defunction the distal bowel and is usually sited in the proximal transverse colon or in the sigmoid colon. A colostomy in the left side of the colon usually produces one to three actions of formed faeces per 24 hours.

The effluent from a transverse colon colostomy resembles that from an ileostomy, being fluid and discharging more or less continuously. It contains proteolytic enzymes and can therefore damage skin; excessive output may cause water and electrolyte depletion.

Permanent End Colostomy

An end colostomy in the sigmoid colon should be sited in the left iliac fossa about half-way between the umbilicus and anterior superior iliac spine centred just medial to the outer border of the rectus abdominis muscle.

Long-Term Management

There are three methods of long-term management.

NATURAL METHOD. Occasionally the colostomy can be relied upon to act at a predictable time each day, often in response to a stimulus such as a hot drink. Between actions a covering such as a plastic cap supported by a belt may be all that is required to maintain cleanliness. Dietary adjustments and drugs such as codeine, loperamide or Lomotil may help to establish this method.

APPLIANCE METHODS. More often, however, the action is not predictable and many patients find a permanent appliance satisfactory. One- or two-piece non-drainable bags are most commonly used, being disposed of and changed after each action. One-piece appliances may be applied to a Stomahesive base which stays in place for several days.

IRRIGATION METHOD. In the irrigation method the colon is emptied by irrigation every 24–48 hours. Advantages include freedom from a bag between irrigations, and perhaps some saving in time and cost. Irrigation should start 2–4 weeks postoperatively under the supervision of a stomatherapist. Kits are commercially available (Holister, Coloplast), and include a short plastic cone, and long plastic sleeve backed by an adhesive flange which fits around the stoma. With the cones now available perforation by an irrigation cannula is no longer a hazard.

The patient sits on the lavatory and connects the cone by tubing to a plastic reservoir suspended at a convenient height. The cone is inserted into the stoma and 750–1000 ml of water at room temperature are run in from the reservoir. A special bag comprising a flange attached to a long plastic sleeve is applied to the stoma and the open end of the sleeve is directed into the lavatory bowl. The colon usually acts after 10–30 minutes and the sleeve is then folded and clipped, enabling the patient to walk around carrying on normal activities during which time a little more effluent escapes. The bag is then removed, the stoma cleaned and a stoma seal applied. If this method is successful colostomy management is quicker, and psychologically more acceptable.

Complications

Severe skin problems are less likely than with an ileostomy but allergy and maceration by moisture resulting from leakage may occur. The remedies are similar to those for ileostomy.

The commonest late complications are paracolostomy hernia, prolapse and stenosis. Hernia is very common and repair is often followed by recurrence. Usually, however, symptoms are minimal and no specific treatment is required. An abdominal support may be necessary if bulging is causing discomfort. Occasionally strangulation occurs and an operation is obligatory. Stenosis and prolapse may require refashioning of the stoma.

Temporary Loop Colostomy

The site for a sigmoid loop colostomy is identical to that for an end colostomy. A transverse loop colostomy should be made through the rectus abdominis muscle away from the costal margin and the abdominal wound.

A loop colostomy requires a permanent appliance which should be drainable if the effluent is liquid. The appliance is larger than is necessary for an end stoma and problems in management of a transverse colostomy are more akin to those of an ileostomy than to a left-sided colostomy.

Appendix B. **Pharmacopoeia**

The following appendix lists a number of drugs commonly used in the treatment of patients with diseases of the colon and rectum. Trade names are given where appropriate as well as the name of the manufacturing company, the active ingredients, and the usual adult dosage.

Approximate prices, quoted in pence, are taken from the most recent editions of the *British National Formulary* (British Medical Association and Pharmaceutical Society of Great Britain) and *Mims* (Medical Publications Ltd). They are intended as a basis for comparison but, because of other factors involved in determining retail prices, may not represent the cost of the dispensed medicine.

Abbreviations

bd	twice daily
tds	three times a daily
qds	four times a day
nocte	at night
IV	intravenous
IM	intramuscular

Anti-inflammatory agents

Steroids

Corticosteroids have been shown to induce remission in active ulcerative colitis and colonic Crohn's disease. They can be given orally, parenterally or topically by suppositories or enemas. Topical administration has the advantage that the drug is directly applied to the area of disease with minimal systemic absorption, but is only suitable for patients with distal disease.

Systemic Preparations (Table B.1)

High doses of steroids may cause cushingoid features and adrenal suppression. Withdrawal of steroids must therefore be by slow reduction to avoid acute adrenal insufficiency. Outpatients taking systemic steroids should carry a card giving details of dosage and possible complications. In children the risks of steroids also include suppression of growth.

Table B.1. Anti-inflammatory agents: Systemic steroids

Name	Active ingredient	Dosage	Cost/day
Tablets			
Prednisolone	Prednisolone	10–60 mg/day	2–12p
Injections			
Codelsol (Merck Sharp & Dohme)	Prednisolone sodium phosphate 16 mg/ml	60 mg/day IV/IM	200p
Delta stab (Boots)	Prednisolone acetate 25 mg/ml	60 mg/day IM	50p
Hydrocortisone	Hydrocortisone sodium succinate	200–400 mg/ day	100–200p

Topical Preparations (Table B.2)

Various steroid preparations are available in the form of suppositories suitable for disease confined to the lower rectum and upper anal canal, or retention enemas that can treat up to the splenic flexure. They should be used after the bowel has been emptied to be retained for as long as possible and are most effective when taken last thing at night. Enemas are best administered with the patient lying on the left side. The lubricated tip of the catheter or disposable applicator is inserted into the anus and the contents slowly injected. The patient should then lie face downwards for 5–10 minutes and try to retain the preparation overnight. Foam formulations are easier to retain but they do not extend as far proximally as liquid enemas. In hospitalised patients hydrocortisone can be given by rectal drip over a period of 30–40 minutes with the patient in bed.

Enemas can be made up by the patient or physician using soluble tablets of prednisolone 21-phosphate (10–40 mg) or betamethasone phosphate (2–4 mg) dissolved in tapwater, to a dose adjusted to the severity of the disease. Such preparations cost only a few pence per day, in contrast to the more expensive commercially available retention enemas.

Table B.2. Anti-inflammatory agents: Topical steroids

Name	Active ingredient	Preparation	Dosage	Cost/ day
Suppositories				
Hydrocortisone	Hydrocortisone acetate	25 mg suppositories	1 bd	40p
Predsol (Glaxo)	Prednisolone sodium phosphate	5 mg suppositories	3 bd	20p
Enemas				
Colifoam (Stafford-Miller)	Hydrocortisone acetate 10%	Foam in aerosol with applicator	1 bd	100p
Proctofoam HC (Stafford-Miller)	Hydrocortisone acetate 1%, pramoxine hydrochloride 1%	Muco-adherent foam in aerosol	1 bd	25p
Cortenema (Bengue)	Hydrocortisone (in viscous suspension)	Retention enema; disposable pack	1 nocte	70p
Predenema (Pharmax)	Prednisolone metasulphobenzoate sodium	Disposable enema pack; long and standard tubes	1 nocte	70– 100p
Predsol (Glaxo)	Prednisolone sodium phosphate 20 mg	Single-dose disposable packs	1 nocte	70p

Sulphasalazine (Table B.3)

Sulphasalazine when used in patients with colonic Crohn's disease and ulcerative colitis has been shown to reduce significantly the likelihood of relapse. It is a combination of 5-amino salicylic acid and sulphapyridine, and is broken down in the caecum by commensal bacteria to release free salicylate. The aspirin component is the active moiety and side effects, which include nausea and vomiting, skin rashes, haematological disorders, photosensitisation and neurotoxicity are due to the sulphonamide component. Sulphasalazine can be given orally, by suppository or retention enema. New delayed-release aspirin preparations have been developed avoiding sulphapyridine as the bound vehicle. Clinical trials are in progress.

Table B.3. Anti-inflammatory agents: Sulphasalazine

Name	Active ingredient	Dosage	Cost/day
Salazopyrin (Pharmacia)	Sulphasalazine	0.5–1 g qds	15–30p
Also available as:			
Enteric coated tablets	Sulphasalazine	0.5–1 g qds	15–30p
Suppositories	Sulphasalazine	0.5–1 g bd	25–30p
Retention enemas	Sulphasalazine	3 g nocte	140p

Azathioprine (Table B.4)

Azathioprine, a derivative of 6-mercaptopurine, is a cytotoxic immunosuppressant that has been used in certain patients with Crohn's disease and ulcerative colitis with the aim of reducing recurrence. There is some evidence in Crohn's disease that it may be effective in preventing relapse and that it can reduce the dose of steroids required to maintain remission.

Azathioprine is toxic to the bone marrow and hepatic toxicity is also recognised. Although the dosage is considerably less than that used after organ transplantation, patients still require careful monitoring with monthly estimation of haemoglobin, white cell and platelet counts when on prolonged treatment.

Table B.4. Anti-inflammatory agents: Azathioprine

Name	Active ingredient	Dosage	Cost/day
Tablets			
Imuran	Azathioprine	50–100 mg tds	100–200p
(Wellcome)			
Azamune	Azathioprine	50–100 mg tds	100–200p
(Penn)			

Laxatives

Laxatives can be divided into four main groups:

  Bulk forming agents
  Osmotic preparations
  Stool softeners and lubricants
  Smooth muscle stimulants

Bulk Forming Agents (Table B.5)

Bulk forming agents work by increasing the faecal mass largely by retaining water. The stool becomes bulky and soft and peristalsis is stimulated. Their action is not immediate and they may take some days to be effective. The patient is encouraged to maintain an adequate fluid intake. Flatulence and abdominal discomfort may occur when the treatment is first started but usually disappear in time and may be dose related.

Table B.5. Laxatives: Bulk forming agents

Name	Active ingredient	Dosage	Cost/day
Unprocessed bran	Bran	12–24 g bd	1p
Fybranta (Norgine)	Bran	1–3 tabs qds	8–24p
Isogel (Allen & Hanburys)	Ispaghula husk	10 ml bd	5p
Fybogel (Reckitt & Coleman)	Ispaghula husk	1 sachet bd	14p
Metamucil (Searle)	Ispaghula husk	1 sachet bd	10p
Celevac (W. B. Pharmaceuticals)	Methylcellulose	3 tabs bd	2–5p
Cologel (Lilly)	Methylcellulose	10–15 ml tds	15–30p
Normacol (Norgine)			
Special	Sterculia		
Standard	Sterculia + frangula	10 ml bd	7–20p
Antispasmodic	Sterculia + alverine citrate		

Osmotic Preparations (Table B.6)

Osmotic preparations act by increasing the volume of fluid within the lumen of the bowel. Taken in large doses they are effective in producing a rapid clearance of the bowel. Saline purgation (by intragastric infusion) is used by many surgeons to prepare the large bowel for surgery. Sodium and water retention can be a problem in the elderly. Mannitol taken by mouth (1 litre 10% in orange juice) is an alternative.

Table B.6. Laxatives: Osmotic preparations

Name	Active ingredients	Dosage	Cost/day
Lactulose (Duphalac, Duphar)	Synthetic disaccharides broken down to acetic and lactic acid	15 ml bd	15–30p
Magnesium hydroxide	Magnesium	5–20 ml bd	1–2p
Magnesium sulphate (Epsom salts)	Magnesium	10–20 ml bd	3–6p
Raes mixture	Magnesium sulphate, liquid paraffin, neostigmine	10–20 ml bd	4–6p
Milpar (Cremaftin) (Boots)	Magnesium hydroxide, liquid paraffin	10–20 ml bd	1–2p

Stool Softeners and Lubricants (Table B.7)

Stool softeners and lubricants may be added to commercial preparations in combination with a stimulant laxative. They have a purely physical effect on the stool.

Table B.7. Laxatives: Stool softeners and lubricants

Name	Active ingredients	Dosage	Cost/day
Dioctyl-Medo (Medo)	Dioctyl sodium sulphosuccinate (docusate)	100 mg bd	3–6p
Liquid paraffin mixture	Liquid paraffin	10–30 ml nocte	2–6p
Petrolagar	Liquid paraffin, light liquid paraffin	10 ml bd	4p

Smooth Muscle Stimulants (Table B.8)

The most commonly used stimulant laxatives are bisacodyl, anthraquinones and senna preparations, which work by increasing intestinal motility via a direct action on smooth muscle. Castor oil works indirectly since it is metabolised by lipolytic enzymes in the small bowel to produce ricinoleic acid which is a colonic irritant. In excessive doses all stimulant laxatives produce abdominal cramps and should not be used in a patient with intestinal obstruction. Prolonged use should be avoided and there is some evidence that permanent damage to the colon may occur. Abuse of stimulant laxatives may cause hypokalaemia. Stimulant laxatives are frequently used for bowel preparation before surgery or X-ray studies. They should be avoided in pregnancy.

Table B.8. Laxatives: Smooth muscle stimulants

Name	Active ingredients	Dosage	Time of action (hours)	Cost/ day
Bisacodyl tablets	Bisacodyl	10 mg nocte	10–12	1–2p
Dulcolax (Boehringer)	Bisacodyl	10 mg nocte	10–12	1–2p
Dulcodos (Boehringer)	Bisacodyl, dioctyl	2 tabs nocte	10–12	2–5p
Cascara tablets	Cascarosides	2 tabs nocte	6–8	1–2p
Castor oil	Metabolised to ricinoleic acid	5–20 ml	2–8	1–5p
Dorbanex (Riker)	Danthron (synthetic anthraquinone)	1–2 capsules	6–12	3–6p

(continued on next page)

Table B.8 *continued*

Name	Active ingredients	Dosage	Time of action (hours)	Cost/day
Normax (Bencard)	Danthron, dioctyl sodium sulpho-succinate	1–3 capsules	6–12	3–6p
Senokot (Reckitt & Colman)	Sennoside	2–4 tabs nocte 5–10 ml syrup nocte	8–12	2–4p
X-Prep[a] (Napp)	Sennoside	71 ml	8–12	50p
Picolax[a] (Nordic)	Sodium picosulphate, magnesium citrate	1 sachet	3	50p

[a] For bowel preparation only.

Rectally Administered Drugs (Table B.9)

Table B.9. Laxatives: Rectally administered drugs

Name	Active ingredients	Cost
Suppositories		
Glycerol	Gelatin; glycerol	4p
Beogex (Pharmax)	Sodium acid phosphate	7p
Dulcolax (Boehringer)	Bisacodyl	5p
Enemas		
Dulcolax (Boehringer)	Bisacodyl solution 2–3 ml	3p
Dioctyl-Medo (Medo)	Faecal softener; docusate 10–40 ml or as elixir with water	10–40p
Fletchers Phosphate enema (Pharmax)	Sodium phosphate, sodium acid phosphate	50p
Micralax micro-enema (SKF)	Sodium citrate, sodium alkylsulphoacetate, sorbic acid	50p
Veripaque (Sterling Research)	Oxyphenisatin	100p

Antidiarrhoeal Drugs

Antidiarrhoeal drugs offer symptomatic relief but do not influence any underlying cause of diarrhoea. They may also be of benefit to the patient with chronic diarrhoea. They can be considered under two broad headings: absorbent mixtures and drugs which reduce bowel motility.

Absorbent Mixtures

Water is absorbed by these agents producing a stool with a more solid consistency. They include kaolin and chalk mixture, and any of the bulking agents listed on p.221.

Drugs which Reduce Bowel Motility (Table B.10)

These drugs act by reducing smooth muscle activity either directly or by parasympathetic autonomic inhibition. Codeine phosphate and loperamide are more effective than diphenoxylate, but codeine being an opiate may produce dependence. Sometimes a combination is necessary to control diarrhoea. The dose should be adjusted to the minimum which produces relief.

Table B.10. Antidiarrhoeal drugs reducing bowel motility

Name	Side effects	Dosage	Cost/day
Codeine phosphate	Nausea, dizziness, sedation, tolerance and dependence	30–60 mg qds	10–25p
Diphenoxylate hydrochloride + atropine (Lomotil) (Gold Cross)	Respiratory depression in children; skin rashes	5 mg qds	50p
Loperamide (Imodium) (Janssen)	Dry mouth, dizziness, headache, skin rashes	2–4 mg qds	80–160p

Antispasmodic Drugs

Antispasmodic drugs may be of use in patients with the irritable bowel syndrome and occasionally in symptomatic diverticular disease. There are two pharmacological types, namely those with anticholinergic effects and those that have a direct effect on smooth muscle.

Anticholinergics (Table B.11)

Anticholinergic agents inhibit parasympathetic activity and therefore reduce secretion and motility of the bowel. Their main disadvantage is that effective therapeutic doses are associated with side effects which include precipitation of glaucoma in elderly patients, visual disturbances, constipation and urinary retention.

Table B.11. Antispasmodic drugs: Anticholinergics

Name	Active ingredient	Dosage	Cost/day
Merbentyl (Merrell)	Dicyclomine hydrochloride	Tabs: 10–20 mg tds Syrup: 10–20 mg	5–10p
Propantheline	Propantheline bromide	15 mg tds	10–15p
Pro-Banthine (Gold Cross)	Propantheline bromide	15–20 mg tds	10–15p

Smooth Muscle Relaxants (Table B.12)

These drugs have a direct relaxant non-anticholinergic effect on intestinal smooth muscle.

Table B.12. Antispasmodic drugs: Smooth muscle relaxants

Name	Active ingredient	Adult dosage	Cost/day
Colofac (Duphar)	Mebeverine hydrochloride	135 mg tds	22p
Colpermin (Tillotts)	Peppermint oil	1–2 capsules tds	30–60p

Antifungal Agents (Table B.13)

The majority of fungal infections affecting the perineal region are due to *Tinea* (ringworm) or *Candida*. Antifungal agents are available as ointments or lotions, the latter being more effective. Dusting powders are available but are therapeutically ineffective. Amphotericin and nystatin are ineffective against *Tinea*.

Table B.13. Antifungal agents

Name	Active ingredient	Cost
Benzoic acid ointment Co (Whitfield's ointment)	Benzoic acid, salicylic acid	25 g 20p
Canestan (Bayer)	Clotrimazole 1%: cream lotion spray	 20 g 100p 20 ml 150p 40 ml 500p

(continued on next page)

Table B.13 *continued*

Name	Active ingredient	Cost
Mycota (Crookes Products)	Zinc undecenoate (cream) Undecenoic acid, dichlorophen (spray)	25 g 50p 110 g 100p
Tineafax (Wellcome)	Zinc undecenoate, naphthenate	25 g 40p
Tinaderm (Kirby-Warrick)	Tolnaftate 1%	15 g 40p
Nystatin (Squibb)	Nystatin 100 000 units/g	15 g 150p
Fungilin (Squibb)	Amphotericin	15 g 140p

Antipruritic Agents (Table B.14)

There is no generally effective antipruritic but topical antihistamines, anaesthetics, emollients and desiccating powders are widely prescribed. Many, however, produce sensitisation of the skin. In the absence of a fungal infection topical steroids may be of value, but should not be used indiscriminately. A barrier cream or powder to protect the skin from moisture is sometimes worthwhile.

Table B.14. Antipruritic agents

Name	Active ingredients	Cost
Soothing agents		
Eurax lotion (Ciba)	Crotamiton 10%	150 ml 140p
Calamine lotion	Calamine, zinc oxide, glycerol, phenol	200 ml 40p
Antihistamines		
Phenergan cream (M & B)	Promethazine	25 g 80p
Anthisan (M & B)	Mepyramine maleate	25 g 80p
Local anaesthetics		
Locan (Duncan Flockhart)	Amethocaine, amylocaine, cinchocaine	30 g 100p
Xylocaine (Astra)	Lignocaine 5%	15 g 70p
Topical steroids		
Hydrocortisone cream	Hydrocortisone acetate 1%	15 g 40p

(continued on next page)

Table B.14 *continued*

Name	Active ingredients	Cost
Cobadex (Cox Pharmaceuticals)	Hydrocortisone, dimethicone	20 g 140p
Emollients, barrier creams		
Zinc and castor oil ointment	Zinc oxide, castor oil	25 g 20p
Vasogen (Pharmax)	Dimethicone, calamine, zinc oxide	50 g 40p
Magnesium hydroxide and phenol lotion	Phenol, zinc oxide, calamine, glycerol, magnesium hydroxide	150 ml 40p
Dusting powders		
Zinc, starch and talc	Zinc oxide, starch, talc	50 g 15p
Talc	Starch 10% sterilised talc	100 g 20p

Topical Applications (Table B.15)

Various preparations are available which have been designed to give symptomatic relief from minor anal and perianal conditions including haemorrhoids and fissure; none has been submitted to controlled clinical trial. They are usually marked both as suppositories and ointments. A local anaesthetic is often incorporated, and the preparation may contain other agents including an astringent, lubricants, vasoconstrictors, a steroid or barrier cream. A few examples are shown in Table B.15.

Table B.15. Topical applications

Name	Type of preparation	Active ingredients	Cost
Anusol (Warner)	Astringent, soothing	Bismuth oxide, zinc oxide	Ointment 25 g 100p Suppos. 1 doz 100p
Anusol HC (Warner)	Astringent, steroid, soothing, antiseptic	Bismuth oxide, hydrocortisone acetate 0.25%, zinc oxide, resorcinol	Ointment 15 g 200p
Anugesic HC (Warner)	Astringent, steroid, surface anaesthetic	Bismuth oxide, hydrocortisone acetate, pramoxine HCl	Ointment 15 g 200p Suppos. 1 doz 200p

(continued on next page)

Table B.15 *continued*

Name	Type of preparation	Active ingredients	Cost
Proctosedyl (Cassenne)	Surface anaesthetic, steroid, antibiotic	Cinchocaine HCl, hydrocortisone, framycetin	Ointment 30 g 500p Suppos. 1 doz 200p
Anodesyn (Crookes Products)	Vasoconstrictor, local anaesthetic, antiseptic	Ephedrine, lignocaine, bronopol	Ointment 25 g 100p Suppos. 1 doz 100p
Lignocaine gel	Surface anaesthetic, antiseptic	Lignocaine HCl 1%, chlorohexidine	15 ml 75p
Xylocaine (Astra)	Antiseptic gel, local anaesthetic	Chlorohexidine, lignocaine HCl 2%	15 ml 75p
Hydrocortisone cream	Steroid	Hydrocortisone acetate 1%	30 g 100p
Cobadex (Cox Pharmaceuticals	Steroid, barrier cream	Hydrocortisone 0.5%, dimethicone 20%	20 g 150p
Vasogen (Pharmax)	Barrier cream, soothing	Dimethicone, calamine, zinc oxide	50 g 50p
Zinc & castor oil ointment	Soothing, barrier cream	Zinc oxide, castor oil, arachis oil	25 g 20p

Subject Index

Colo-Proctology

Edited by **J.-C. Givel, F. Saegesser**
1984. 85 figures, 66 tables. XII, 182 pages
ISBN 3-540-12557-4

The 1983 Anglo-Swiss Colo-Proctology Meeting, whose proceedings are contained in this volume, enabled numerous specialists to share their experiences in lower gastrointestinal tract pathology. The focus was on ischaemic disease and tumours of the colon, rectum and anus. The articles are written by international authorities in their field, and several contain unpublished results which may lead to new diagnostic and therapeutic methods.
Ischaemic lesions are considered in this work because they are far more common than is recognised on clinical grounds alone, particularly in the gastrointestinal tract. Large intestine ischaemia is often confused with other syndromes, especially since the clinical features evoked are, in most cases, atypical. Thus diagnosis is frequently late with dramatic consequences.
The oncology chapter treats basically the early diagnosis of gastrointestinal tumours – a prerequisite for improving survival in affected patients – and also presentation and treatment of certain rare tumours.
The third section of this volume covers diverse subjects such as surgical technique, functional disorders of the large intestine, inflammatory bowel disease, haemorrhoids and investigatory procedures.

A. Huber, A. H. C. v. Hochstetter, M. Allgöwer

Transsphincteric Surgery of the Rectum

Topographical Anatomy and Operation Technique

Translated from the German by T. C. Telger
1984. 31 figures, most in color, in 58 separate illustrations.
VII, 83 pages. ISBN 3-540-13050-0

This atlas illustrates and describes the topographical anatomy of planned transsphincteric approaches and operative technique. In contrast to the familiar surgical texts, here the anatomical principles are expounded on the basis of accurate preparations of the individual elements of the anorectum, and vasculature, innervation and the functional relations involved in the preservation of continence are shown. Attention is drawn to improvements achieved as a result of the anatomical studies and to the mastering of technical difficulties. Finally, with the aid of many examples of the author's own cases, indications and clinical experience with this operative technique are presented and discussed.
The impressive color illustrations, prepared by A. Huber, are without equal. Every surgeon will greet this volume as an indispensable work of reference.

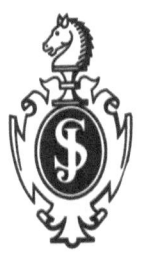

Springer-Verlag
Berlin
Heidelberg
New York
Tokyo

Comprehensive Manuals of Surgical Specialties

A Springer Series
Edited by
Richard H. Egdahl

C. E. Welch, L. W. Ottinger, J. P. Welch

Manual of Lower Gastrointestinal Surgery

Illustrated by **E. Tagrin** and **R. J. Galla**
1980. 215 figures (138 in color), 7 tables.
XVI, 276 pages. ISBN 3-540-90205-8

"It is not often that a surgical text is published representing, as it were, the lifetime experience of an accomplished senior surgeon. Claude Welch and coauthors have given us such a volume in their **Manual of Lower Gastrointestinal Surgery.** Looking back over the years, he gives the reader a perspective that is unique in its objectivity yet, at the same time, extremely helpful in answering the everyday questions that confront a practising surgeon."

Surgery, Gynecology and Obstetrics

Manual of Ambulatory Surgery

Edited by **K. J. Kassity, J. E. McKittrick,** and **F. W. Preston**
Illustrated by **J. C. Koelling**
1982. 270 figures (172 in full color).
XVIII, 266 pages. ISBN 3-540-90700-9

"The recent growth of ambulatory surgery ... is underscored by the publication of this beautiful book, which elegantly describes the administrative and surgical techniques used in a well-established, hospital-based ambulatory surgical center ... The book is printed on durable, glossy paper with large, readable type and generous margins, as befits a manual that should withstand years of use in a busy operating room. It should be available in every surgical suite..."

The New England Journal of Medicine

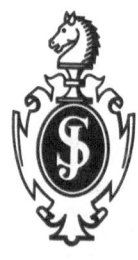

Springer-Verlag
Berlin
Heidelberg
New York
Tokyo